BLOOD TESTS
MADE EASY

BLOOD TESTS
MADE EASY

Paul Hamilton, BSc (Hons), MB BCh BAO (Hons), PGDipToxicol, PGCCE, MD, FRCP (Edin), FRCPath

Clinical Lecturer
Centre for Medical Education
Queen's University Belfast;
Consultant Chemical Pathologist
Belfast Health and Social Care Trust
Belfast, UK

ELSEVIER

Notices

Practitioners and researchers must always rely on their own experience and knowledge in evaluating and using any information, methods, compounds or experiments described herein. Because of rapid advances in the medical sciences, in particular, independent verification of diagnoses and drug dosages should be made. To the fullest extent of the law, no responsibility is assumed by Elsevier, authors, editors or contributors for any injury and/or damage to persons or property as a matter of products liability, negligence or otherwise, or from any use or operation of any methods, products, instructions, or ideas contained in the material herein.

ISBN: 978-0-3238-7044-3
Printed in India
Last digit is the print number: 9 8 7 6 5 4 3 2 1

Content Strategist: Trinity Hutton
Content Project Manager: Arindam Banerjee
Design: Patrick C. Ferguson
Illustration Manager: Akshaya Mohan
Marketing Manager: Deborah Watkins

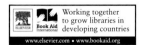

Contents

Preface

The majority of decisions relating to diagnosis and treatment in medicine, centre around the correct interpretation of a laboratory test result. However, there is evidence that suggests that newly qualified doctors and other healthcare professionals often lack sufficient skills in interpreting these data. Traditional texts dealing with this subject are often viewed by students as being complicated and lengthy, focusing on physiology or pathophysiology rather than on the interpretation of the test results themselves. For example, someone reading about acute pancreatitis will learn that amylase is a useful test to perform and when studying hyperaldosteronism, the reader will learn that this condition lowers potassium. Whilst these are undoubtedly useful pieces of information, it is also extremely important to be able to think about amylase and potassium in their own rights and to consider other causes of abnormalities in these results. This is a particularly important skill for doctors who are responsible for checking blood results for entire wards of patients, some of whom will be unfamiliar to the doctor. Often, the last task of the working day is to scan through lots of blood results. Finding a significant abnormality can sometimes be a cause for anxiety.

I hope that this book will be useful to medical students and newly qualified doctors. I also hope that this book will help nurses, biomedical scientists, clinical scientists and anyone else who is required to interpret laboratory results.

This book is written from the viewpoint of a practising chemical pathologist who used to work as a consultant physician in acute and general medicine. The guidance provided is practical and pragmatic, rather than all-inclusive and overly detailed. When causes of abnormalities are listed in this book, I have tended to include the most common conditions, rather than exhaustive lists. Mastery of the basics sets a good foundation for later development. Interested readers should turn to larger reference texts if they are willing to explore a particular test in more detail.

Paul Hamilton, UK

Using this book

You will note that no reference ranges have been provided in the book. This is because such values vary from laboratory to laboratory, and it is always important to use reference ranges provided by the laboratory for the particular test you are interpreting.

The majority of information provided in this book relates to adult patients. Where a topic is of particular relevance to paediatric patients, some guidance has been provided. Whilst much of what is said is applicable to children, readers are encouraged to exercise caution in this regard.

There are no chapters on the interpretation of blood results in relation to infection. This is simply because the laboratory reports that stem from such requests are usually self-explanatory. The general principles outlined in the early chapters remain valid when it comes to requesting such tests.

Only blood tests are considered in this book but bear in mind that the analysis of other bodily fluids (e.g., urine, cerebrospinal fluid) can be extremely helpful and sometimes essential in making a diagnosis.

Dedication

This book is dedicated to the memory of my Dad, Raymond Hamilton.
I hope that some of his ability to explain complicated things in simple ways
rubbed off on me.

Effective use of laboratory tests

SELECTING APPROPRIATE TESTS

Theoretically, you could order every test in this book for every patient you come across. The advantage of this approach is that you would probably diagnose the patient's problem without too much thought (assuming that the responsible diagnosis could be made from or suggested by a blood test). However, this practice would:

- require a large volume of blood
- cost a lot of money
- overwhelm the laboratory
- generate some 'abnormal' results that are irrelevant and that may lead to further investigations and patient anxiety.

Tests should be chosen with a particular purpose in mind, and ideally with an appreciation of what impact a result might have on management. Some tests are inexpensive to perform and yield information about conditions which can have non-specific symptoms. These are considered general screening tests, are requested very frequently and include the urea and

1

electrolyte profile (see Chapter 3) and the full blood picture (see Chapter 15). In some institutions, laboratories and clinicians have collaborated and agreed on 'panels' of blood tests which are helpful in certain situations, e.g., an 'abdominal pain' panel that might include tests such as amylase/ lipase, liver enzymes and C-reactive protein.

MAIN LABORATORY VS POINT-OF-CARE TESTING (POCT)

POCT involves the analysis of a sample in the patient's vicinity (e.g., in a GP's surgery or on a hospital ward), rather than transporting a sample to a large, central laboratory. The most common point-of-care blood tests are capillary blood glucose monitors and blood gas analysis. POCT has advantages and disadvantages.

Advantages of POCT

- improved speed of analysis
- reduced administration
- helpful for remote areas
- quick and easy to repeat a test

Disadvantages of POCT

- all operators must be trained and competence maintained
- errors if machines are not maintained properly
- extra work for the requestor

LABORATORY ASSAY METHODOLOGY

To many requestors of blood tests, laboratories are mysterious places where blood samples enter and, after some time, results are released. Whilst it is not essential for most professionals to understand the full details of sample analysis, appreciation of some broad principles should be helpful, particularly in understanding some of the limitations of laboratory testing. The main techniques in frequent use are as follows.

Chromatography

A technique for separating mixtures into their constituent components. There are several methods in use, including liquid and gas chromatography. Samples are loaded into the device and the contents separate out depending on their characteristics. A detector and recorder are used to record a series of peaks which correspond to what is in the sample.

Commonly used for: toxic alcohols.
Comments: manual interpretation of traces is required, not suitable for high-throughput testing.

Electrophoresis

Constituents within a sample are separated based on differences in how they move in a medium when an electric current is applied.
Commonly used for: investigation of proteins in serum.
Comments: manual interpretation of traces is required, so not suitable for high-throughput testing.

Flow cytometry

The sample is injected through a laser beam and the particular way in which the light is scattered is used to identify the cells present.
Commonly used for: full blood picture.

Immunoassay

Specially designed antibodies are introduced into a sample. These attach to the substance under investigation. Various techniques are then used to detect the antibody-antigen complex.
Commonly used for: troponin, C-reactive protein.
Common problems: Heterophilic antibodies are antibodies already present in a sample that interfere with the expected binding of the testing antibodies, meaning that spurious results are obtained. The 'high dose hook' effect is the name given to the production of a falsely low result in a patient whose true result is very high.

Potentiometry

Specially designed ion-specific electrodes that respond to the particular substance being measured are introduced into the sample. A change in the electrical signal detected corresponds to the concentration of the substance in the sample.
Commonly used for: sodium, potassium.
Common problems: pseudohyponatraemia (see Chapter 3 for details).

Mass spectrometry

This is a very sophisticated technique in which constituents of a sample are fragmented. Fragments have very specific characteristics that allow them

3

to be identified. Mass spectrometry is often coupled with chromatography: chromatography being used to separate the constituents of a sample and mass spectrometry used to identify them.
Commonly used for: therapeutic drug monitoring, some hormones.
Comments: not suitable for high-throughput testing.

Microscopy

The sample is placed on a glass slide and examined under a microscope.
Commonly used for: blood film interpretation.

Spectrophotometry

This technique measures the amount of light that is absorbed as it passes through a sample, often after a dye has been added.
Commonly used for: calcium, magnesium.

Osmometry

This technique is used to estimate the number of osmotically active particles in a solution. 'Freezing point depression' is one variant of this in which the freezing point of a sample is determined and used to estimate the osmolality of the solution.
Commonly used for: osmolality.

Interpreting laboratory tests

SAMPLE TYPES

There are three main sample types used for blood tests. These are illustrated in Fig. 2.1 and described below:

1. Whole blood. Blood is drawn from an artery or vein, mixed with an anticoagulant in a special syringe or tube, and injected into an analyser. This is the most common specimen type for haematological testing and for POCT.
2. Serum. Blood is drawn into a bottle which has a chemical inside to accelerate clotting. The clotted blood is then centrifuged in the laboratory. The straw-coloured liquid that settles at the top of the bottle is serum. Serum is blood minus the cells and clotting factors.
3. Plasma. Blood is drawn into a bottle which has a chemical inside to prevent clotting. The sample is then centrifuged in the laboratory. The straw-coloured liquid that settles at the top of the bottle is plasma. Plasma is blood minus the cells.

Practitioners should consult with their local laboratory to learn the particular sample type for the test they are requesting. Reference ranges

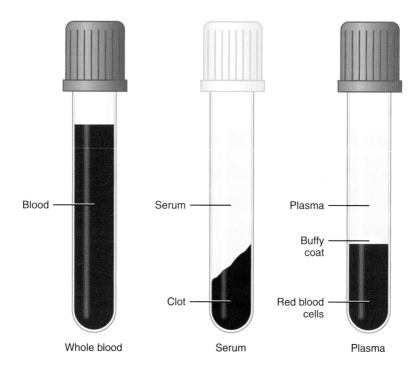

Fig. 2.1 *The difference between whole blood, serum and plasma*

should also be consulted, as they often differ depending on the type of sample that is analysed.

LABORATORY REPORTS

Reports will look different depending on the system in use by any particular laboratory. Reports may be issued on paper or electronically. Most blood test reports have similar constituent parts as shown in Fig. 2.2.

Always take time to check that the report that you are looking at corresponds to the patient in question.

REFERENCE RANGES

A reference range (often incorrectly called a 'normal range') enables us to decide if a particular result is unusual or fairly similar to most other comparable people. One way that laboratories go about this process is by testing a large number of people in the population to see what the test result is for them. These results are then plotted and a graph, similar to that shown

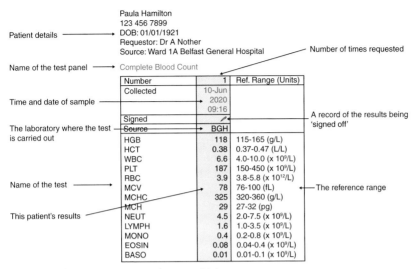

Patient details

Name of the test panel

Time and date of sample

The laboratory where the test is carried out

Name of the test

This patient's results

Number of times requested

A record of the results being 'signed off'

The reference range

Paula Hamilton
123 456 7899
DOB: 01/01/1921
Requestor: Dr A Nother
Source: Ward 1A Belfast General Hospital

Complete Blood Count

	Number	1	Ref. Range (Units)
	Collected	10-Jun 2020 09:16	
	Signed		
	Source	BGH	
	HGB	118	115-165 (g/L)
	HCT	0.38	0.37-0.47 (L/L)
	WBC	6.6	4.0-10.0 (x 10⁹/L)
	PLT	187	150-450 (x 10⁹/L)
	RBC	3.9	3.8-5.8 (x 10¹²/L)
	MCV	78	76-100 (fL)
	MCHC	325	320-360 (g/L)
	MCH	29	27-32 (pg)
	NEUT	4.5	2.0-7.5 (x 10⁹/L)
	LYMPH	1.6	1.0-3.5 (x 10⁹/L)
	MONO	0.4	0.2-0.8 (x 10⁹/L)
	EOSIN	0.08	0.04-0.4 (x 10⁹/L)
	BASO	0.01	0.01-0.1 (x 10⁹/L)

Fig. 2.2 *The constituent parts of a typical laboratory report*

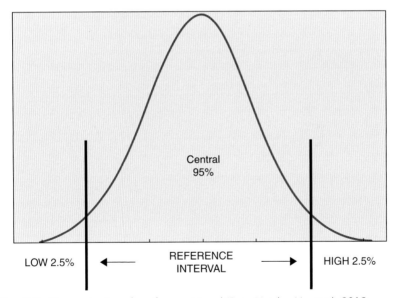

Central
95%

LOW 2.5%   REFERENCE INTERVAL   HIGH 2.5%

Fig. 2.3 *The construction of a reference interval (From Murphy, M., et al. 2019. Clinical Biochemistry: An Illustrated Colour Text, 6th Edition.)*

in Fig. 2.3, will be generated. Most people will have a result that centres around some sort of average value. As we go further and further from the average, fewer and fewer people will have such a result. If we set limits on the results as shown by the bars in the figure, we can define a central area

7

in which 95% of results will fall. This is how reference intervals are set. It follows then, for many tests, that 2.5% of people in the population will have a result above any particular reference range, and 2.5% will have a result below it. A result outside the reference range does not therefore mean that a patient is abnormal, and a result inside the reference range does not mean that a patient is normal. The further away a result is from the reference range, the more likely it becomes that the patient is significantly different from the healthy population.

Reference ranges can be affected by a range of factors particular to the test in question. Table 2.1 gives some examples. Always ensure that you are interpreting results by comparing to an appropriate reference range.

Factor	Example
Age	Alkaline phosphatase in a growing teenager is generally much higher than that in an adult, due to bone growth
Sex	The reference range for testosterone is much higher in an adult male than an adult female
Time	Cortisol levels are generally higher on waking than just before sleeping
Recent activity	Glucose will rise after a sugary snack
Pregnancy	Uric acid levels tend to rise in late pregnancy
Body composition	Amputees will have lower creatinine levels than people with all four limbs
Posture	Renin levels tend to rise on standing up

Table 2.1 *Examples of common factors which can influence a laboratory test result*

Cut-off values or decision levels

For some results, practitioners will compare measured results to a particular cut-off value rather than a reference range. Such decision levels are usually chosen by a group of experts to maximise the usefulness of a test after due consideration of its performance characteristics. When using such values to make decisions, bear in mind that no test is 100% sensitive and 100% specific, and that there will always be the chance of a false positive or false negative. These concepts are explored further in Chapter 11.

TRENDS

Trends in results are generally much more useful than one-off results. Take Fig. 2.4 as an example.

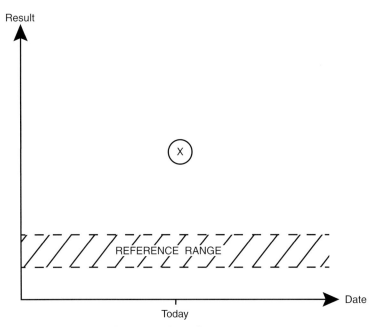

Fig. 2.4 *Interpreting one-off results is often difficult*

The test in question could be a marker of infection or a tumour marker, for example. A one-off result higher than the reference range would be a cause for concern. If the result is taken in the context of previous results, however, it becomes much more meaningful as shown in Fig. 2.5.

PATTERNS OF RESULTS

The human brain is good at spotting patterns. This can prove very helpful when it comes to blood test interpretation. Patterns will be highlighted at appropriate sections in the book, but the Table 2.2 illustrates some classical patterns.

Pattern	One possible explanation
Low haemoglobin with extremely low mean cell volume	Thalassaemia
Low sodium with high potassium	Hypoadrenalism
Low potassium with high total carbon dioxide	Vomiting
Very high alkaline phosphatase and gamma glutamyl transpeptidase	Cholestasis
Various classical abnormalities – see next section	Sample contamination

Table 2.2 *Characteristic patterns of results*

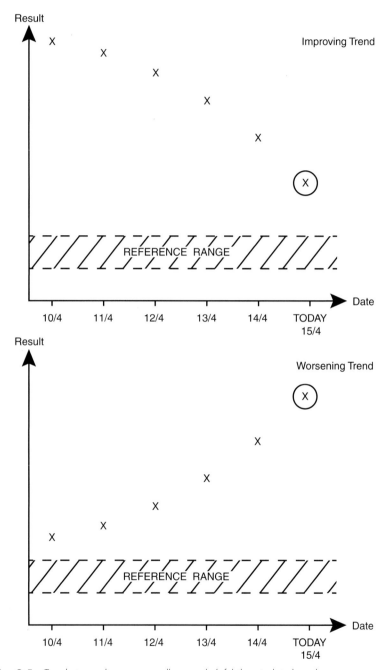

Fig. 2.5 *Trends in results are generally more helpful than isolated results*

PROBLEM SAMPLES

Haemolysis

If venepuncture is particularly traumatic, or if a sample is not handled carefully, the red blood cells in the blood can rupture (haemolyse). Haemolysis can also occur inside the body by a variety of mechanisms such as autoimmune disease or mechanical rupture by prosthetic heart valves. The contents of the red cells will then spill out, and erroneous values for some tests will be obtained if these contents are analysed (see Table 2.3). Additionally, the colour of serum or plasma will become more red than normal after haemolysis, and this can affect the measurement of other components.

Potassium
Lactate dehydrogenase
Aspartate aminotransferase
Bilirubin
Alanine aminotransferase
Gamma glutamyl transpeptidase
Phosphate
Ammonia
Magnesium

Table 2.3   *Tests commonly affected by haemolysis*

Although laboratories always test for haemolysis in samples and do not report affected results (you will see comments such as "Haemolysis present; no result available"), such checks are not performed by most POCT devices, and results are released without warning.

Contaminated samples

If a patient has an intravenous infusion running into an intravenous catheter located in the dorsum of the hand, blood taken from the antecubital fossa from the same limb will be contaminated by the infusion. Dilute fluids will cause falsely low values for some results while infused electrolytes, for example, will cause spuriously high results. Drug infusions can also occasionally interfere with results, e.g., patients with dopamine infusions can have falsely low measures of creatinine because of an interference between dopamine and a common laboratory assay used in creatinine measurement.

Wrong patient identifier

When sending a sample to a laboratory, always ensure that you have completed the necessary sections of the request form, otherwise your sample may be rejected due to inadequate labelling. Occasionally a sample is mislabelled at source, and this can cause results which are totally out of keeping for a patient, as illustrated in Fig. 2.6. If the results that you are looking at are completely unexpected, always repeat the sample.

Incorrect blood tube in use

There are a wide variety of blood tubes available, and the correct tube must always be used for the test being requested. Several tube types are prepared with a chemical inside the tube, and the colour of the cap indicates the type of tube. Tubes in common use in the UK (made by BD, Franklin Lakes, USA) are shown in Table 2.4.

Some of the chemicals in use can interfere with common tests, e.g., lithium will be high in any sample collected in a lithium-heparin tube, so correct tube choice is a must. Additionally, it is important that when taking blood into multiple tubes, the practitioner follows the correct 'order of draw' to minimise the chance of a chemical from a previous tube interfering with tests in the next tube. If a needle is used to transfer blood into an EDTA tube and then is used to transfer blood to a gel separator tube, for example, a small amount of EDTA will end up in the second tube and cause interference. Common interferences are highlighted in Table 2.5.

Date	1st January	2nd January	3rd January	4th January	5th January	5th January
Time	09:00	09:00	09:00	09:00	09:00	11:00
Sodium (mmol/L)	140	141	139	139	142	141
Potassium (mmol/L)	3.5	3.5	3.5	3.6	5.8	3.5
Chloride (mmol/L)	99	98	100	97	102	98
Total CO_2 (mmol/L)	26	25	26	26	20	25
Urea (mmol/L)	5.2	4.8	5.0	5.1	18.7	5.1
Creatinine (μmol/L)	51	56	49	55	492	57
eGFR (mL/min/1.73 m²)	>60	>60	>60	>60	9	>60

Results generally similar over a period of 4 days.

Marked change in some results. The blood sample belongs to a different patient, but has been incorrectly labelled.

The correct results for the patient.

Fig. 2.6 *An illustration of the value of always interpreting results in context*

Tube cap colour	Chemical in tube	Common uses
Light blue	Sodium citrate	Coagulation testing
Gold	Gel separator	Urea and electrolytes
Red	-	Drug levels
Green	Lithium-Heparin	Ethylene glycol
Purple	Potassium-EDTA	Full blood picture
Pink	Potassium-EDTA	Blood grouping
Grey	Sodium fluoride	Glucose

Table 2.4 *Blood collection tubes in common use in the UK*

Chemical causing problem	Common effects
Sodium citrate	Raises sodium (a good clue is a simultaneous unusually low chloride) Lowers calcium
Potassium-EDTA	Raises potassium Lowers calcium, magnesium and alkaline phosphatase

Table 2.5 *Common interference patterns in biochemical results*

MINIMAL SIGNIFICANT CHANGE

If 40 mL of blood is taken from a patient, split into ten 4 mL tubes and analysed for a particular test, it is highly unlikely that exactly the same result will arise on all ten occasions. The results will all cluster around a mean result due to analytical variation. Similarly, if 4 mL of blood is taken from the same patient on ten consecutive days at the same time each day and under the same conditions, ten slightly different results would be expected because of biological variation.

If a patient has a serum sodium concentration of 120 mmol/L at 9 a.m. and 121 mmol/L at 12 p.m., does that represent an improvement or simply the effects of variation? To answer this question, one must consider both analytical and biological variation for the test in question. Such data are available in reference text books or from your laboratory.

CHAPTER 3

Osmolality and the urea and electrolyte (U+E) profile

OUTLINE

OSMOLALITY

Osmolality is a measure of the number of particles in a solution. It provides no information about the nature of the particles. Consider Fig. 3.1.

The key 'particles' in blood in terms of osmolality are sodium, urea and glucose. Abnormalities in osmolality results are generally due to issues with these substances as shown in Table 3.1.

If osmolality in extracellular fluid changes, water will move across cell membranes in an attempt to equalise osmolality. Major problems can ensue when this happens in the brain, as shown below. Expansion of the brain inside the hard confines of the skull can have fatal consequences for a patient as depicted simplistically in Fig. 3.2.

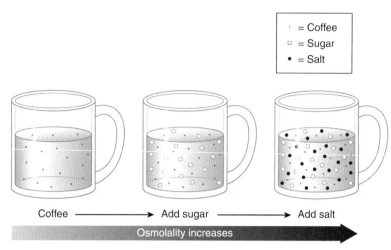

Fig. 3.1 *Increasing osmolality in a cup of coffee*

Low Osmolality	High Osmolality
Hyponatraemia	Hypernatraemia
	Hyperglycaemia
	Ingested substances e.g., toxic alcohols

Table 3.1 *Common causes of abnormal blood osmolality*

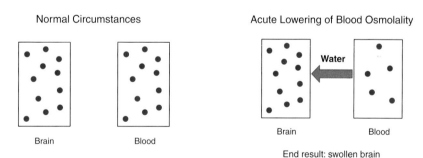

Fig. 3.2 *How an acute drop in blood osmolality can cause brain swelling*

You may come across the term 'osmolarity' which is technically different to 'osmolality', but for most purposes in medicine, the two terms can be considered broadly similar. The terms should not be used interchangeably.

Osmolar gap

Osmolality is measured in the laboratory, but an estimate of osmolality can be calculated using the following formula (when all results are in mmol/L):

Calculated osmolality = 2 × (Sodium + Potassium) + Urea + Glucose

If the measured osmolality is different to the calculated osmolality, an osmolar gap is present. The higher the gap, the more likely it is that the patient has an unidentified osmotically active substance in their system. Calculating the osmolar gap is most useful in patients who have taken a toxic alcohol in an attempt at self-harm, e.g., ethylene glycol. The level of gap that is significant is often disputed, but a gap of 10 or more is likely to be significant. If you identify a high osmolar gap, try to work out what osmotically active substance is responsible.

CORE COMPONENTS OF THE UREA AND ELECTROLYTE (U+E) PROFILE

A U+E profile typically comprises measures of sodium, potassium, total carbon dioxide, chloride, urea, and creatinine.

SODIUM

Sodium is the most abundant cation in blood and, as such, is the major contributor to osmolality. Problems that arise because of hypo- or hyper-natraemia happen because of changes to the osmolality of the blood.

If a blood sample has large amounts of protein (e.g., in a patient with multiple myeloma) or triglyceride (e.g., in a patient with a genetic lipid disorder), a falsely low sodium result may be returned when the same is analysed in the main laboratory. This is pseudohyponatraemia. Due to a difference in the way that the analysis is run, a true sodium result will be obtained when the same sample is tested in a POCT analyser. Osmolality should always be checked in cases of hyponatraemia. In true hyponatraemia, osmolality will be low. In pseudohyponatraemia, osmolality will be normal.

Hyponatraemia

Consider the glass of salty water in Fig. 3.3.
The concentration of sodium in the glass can be decreased by:
1. adding water
2. removing both sodium and water, but proportionally more sodium
3. removing sodium and leaving the volume of water unchanged

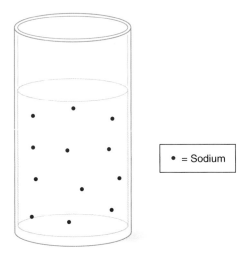

Fig. 3.3 *A glass of salty water*

The sodium concentration in blood can be decreased by similar means, although the last option is uncommon.

There are three key questions to ask when dealing with hyponatraemia:

1. Is it really hyponatraemia? Check osmolality as detailed above.
2. Is the hyponatraemia an emergency? Two factors constitute a hyponatraemia emergency requiring urgent intervention:
   a. Hyponatraemia of rapid onset. A large drop occurring quickly does not give the brain cells time to adapt to the sudden drop in osmolality.
   b. Hyponatraemia accompanied by features of cerebral oedema, e.g., headache, nausea, vomiting, confusion, seizures, depressed level of consciousness.
3. What is the fluid status of the patient? Establishing if the patient is volume deplete (i.e. dehydrated), volume neutral (i.e. euvolaemic) or volume overloaded will help establish the cause of the hyponatraemia and plan treatment. A careful clinical examination is necessary, as is inspection of any fluid-balance charts. Testing the concentration of sodium in the urine can also be helpful.

Using the information above, one can begin to ascertain the cause for the hyponatraemia and plan appropriate treatment. Common causes are listed in Table 3.2.

Volume depleted	Volume neutral	Volume overloaded
Vomiting	Syndrome of inappropriate	Heart failure
Diarrhoea	ADH (SIADH)*	Liver failure
Diuretics	Primary polydipsia	Renal failure
Salt wasting states		
Hypoadrenalism		

*SIADH (syndrome of inappropriate antidiuretic hormone secretion) itself has a large number of causes and is a diagnosis of exclusion. In particular, hypoadrenalism, hypothyroidism, renal failure and hypopituitarism should be excluded before this diagnosis is made.

Table 3.2 *Common causes of hyponatraemia*

Hypernatraemia

Thinking about the glass of salty water from Fig. 3.3 again, the concentration of sodium in the glass can be increased by:
1. adding sodium
2. removing both sodium and water, but proportionally more water
3. removing water and leaving the amount of sodium unchanged

Although the sodium concentration in blood can be increased by similar means, the second option is by far the commonest mechanism. This tends to occur most commonly in elderly patients who are unable to drink adequate water for their requirements.

Option 3 describes what happens in diabetes insipidus, a condition in which a patient passes excessively dilute urine which can be picked up by testing urinary osmolality. Healthy people who are rendered hypernatraemic tend to pass very concentrated urine. If the urine is inappropriately dilute, diabetes insipidus is a possibility. Further coverage of this condition is provided in Chapter 7.

POTASSIUM

As detailed in Chapter 2, haemolysis of a sample will spuriously raise the measured potassium. This is usually very apparent when samples are analysed in a main laboratory, as it is common practice to check for the presence of haemolysis on all samples prior to checking potassium. A haemolysed sample that passes through a main laboratory analyser will usually be reported as 'Sample haemolysed; no result available.' When whole blood potassium is analysed on a point-of-care device however, no haemolysis checks are performed. If the sample is haemolysed, the results given will be falsely elevated.

Abnormalities in potassium cause problems with neuromuscular function, and in particular cardiac conduction. Hyperkalaemia is a medical emergency.

When considering problems relating to potassium, you might find the concepts shown in Fig. 3.4 and Fig. 3.5 helpful.

Most of the body's potassium is inside cells. View these as a kind of store for potassium. With this concept in mind, hypo- and hyperkalaemia can each be considered under three headings: too little or too much coming in; a shift into or out of the store; and too much or too little going out. It is much easier to remember these general principles and then some causes for each, than a long list of random causes. When it comes to renal losses of potassium, remember that the hormone aldosterone normally functions to get potassium out of the body.

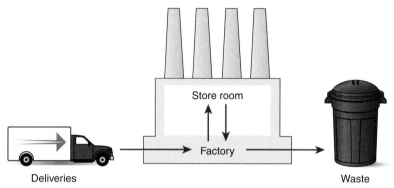

Fig. 3.4 *A simple model of a factory which can assist in understanding some electrolyte abnormalities*

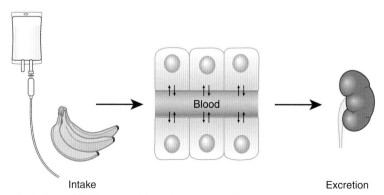

Fig. 3.5 *A simplified version of how the body handles potassium*

Too little in	Chronic malnutrition
	'Nil by mouth' with inadequate replacement
Shift from blood into cells	Alkalosis
	Re-feeding syndrome
	Drugs, e.g., salbutamol, insulin
Too much out	Hyperaldosteronism
	Diuretics
	Diarrhoea, vomiting

Table 3.3 *Common causes of hypokalaemia*

Hypokalaemia

Common causes of hypokalaemia are shown in Table 3.3.

Hyperkalaemia

Spurious causes for hyperkalaemia (sometimes called pseudohyperkalaemia) are particularly common, and include:

- Haemolysis: this will be detected and reported if the sample is analysed in a main laboratory but neither detected nor reported on a point-of-care machine. Because the concentration of potassium is high inside cells, any cell breakdown will falsely raise the measured level.
- Delayed sample processing (e.g., when a sample is transported to a laboratory from a remote general practitioner's surgery). The potassium slowly leaks out of cells – the longer it takes to test the sample, the more that leaks out.
- Contaminated sample (see Chapter 2).
- Prolonged application of a tourniquet when taking blood (again, due to leak of potassium out of cells 'trapped' in the occluded vein).
- Excessive fist clenching during venepuncture (potassium leaks out of the muscles).
- Thrombocytosis (e.g., patients with essential thrombocytosis and a grossly elevated platelet count), potassium leaks out of platelets.
- Leucocytosis (e.g., patients with leukaemia), potassium leaks out of leucocytes.
- Genuine causes of hyperkalaemia are shown in Table 3.4.

TOTAL CARBON DIOXIDE (AND BICARBONATE)

Total CO_2 represents the total amount of bicarbonate ions, dissolved CO_2 and other CO_2-containing substances in a solution. Since bicarbonate

Too much in	Overzealous IV replacement
Shift from blood	Acidosis
into cells	Tissue damage, e.g., rhabdomyolysis
Too little out	Kidney failure (acute or chronic)
	Hypoaldosteronism
	Drugs, e.g., ACE-inhibitors, angiotensin receptor blockers, potassium-sparing diuretics

Table 3.4 *Common causes of hyperkalaemia*

normally constitutes the majority of this, total CO_2 is usually used as a convenient surrogate measure of bicarbonate, as it is much easier to measure in the laboratory than bicarbonate per se. The total CO_2 on the electrolyte profile may provide the first clue to the presence of an acid-base disturbance in a patient.

Low level: a metabolic acidosis is likely to be present as bicarbonate is being used up, as it buffers excess acid in the body.

High level: a metabolic alkalosis is likely to be present.

If an acid-base disorder is suspected, testing of pH and blood gases is required to enable a full assessment (see Chapter 6 for details).

CHLORIDE

Abnormalities in chloride typically follow those in sodium. Thus, low concentrations of chloride typically accompany hyponatraemia and high concentrations in hypernatraemia. If a high sodium concentration and low chloride concentration are noted, you should suspect sodium citrate contamination of the specimen (see Chapter 2 for details). Chloride results are necessary when calculating an anion gap (see Chapter 6 for details).

UREA

Urea is principally a by-product of protein metabolism in the liver. It is filtered at the glomeruli and can be reabsorbed in the kidney tubules. Reabsorption is particularly noticeable in states of dehydration. Knowledge of these key facts should help you interpret abnormal urea results. Common causes for urea abnormalities are shown in Table 3.5.

CREATININE

Creatinine is a waste product formed in muscles, and is a commonly used test to provide some information about glomerular filtration rate (GFR), a key measure of kidney function. The baseline creatinine concentration in a

Low urea	High urea
Malnutrition Liver disease	Tissue catabolism (e.g., patients with critical illness) – due to increased protein breakdown High protein intake Gastrointestinal tract haemorrhage (blood contents are digested in the gut) Dehydration Renal disease

Table 3.5 *Common causes of an abnormal urea concentration*

person with healthy kidneys is mainly determined by their muscle mass, and so will be much higher in a weightlifter than in an inactive elderly person. If one is simply considering a blood test in isolation, the composition of the patient will not be known. A result that might be considered normal for the weightlifter will be very abnormal for the older person. It is therefore most useful to look back on old creatinine levels in a patient to compare current to previous. If someone's creatinine is normally around 50 µmol/L but is now 100 µmol/L, their GFR is likely to have fallen considerably, even though the creatinine level may still be within the reference range of the laboratory. For this reason, creatinine concentrations are most useful when viewed in the context of previous results. To get around this difficulty, estimated GFR is usually calculated.

ESTIMATED GLOMERULAR FILTRATION RATE (EGFR)

Because of the limitations of creatinine measurement in terms of estimating glomerular filtration rate (GFR), a standardised 'estimated' GFR is often calculated by laboratories. There are several formulae in current use which utilise creatinine with other information such as age, sex, ethnicity, urea and albumin concentration, in an attempt to more accurately estimate GFR. Because creatinine concentrations are dependent on both muscle mass and GFR, a result of 120 µmol/L might be found in a bodybuilder with healthy kidneys but, if present in a short, thin, elderly person, would indicate significant renal impairment. If a patient has chronic kidney disease, it is standard practice to classify that disease on the basis of GFR and urinary albumin excretion.

ACUTE KIDNEY INJURY E-ALERTS

Modern laboratory information systems often employ an algorithm that compares current creatinine results to historical values. If a series of conditions are met, an electronic alert is often attached to the laboratory result. The higher the alert grade (1, 2 or 3), the more marked is the change in creatinine.

The bone profile

CALCIUM

Understanding abnormal calcium results requires knowledge of several connected physiological pathways, shown in Fig. 4.1. The body's main store of calcium is the skeleton. When circulating calcium levels fall, para-thyroid hormone (PTH) is released from the parathyroid glands and works to raise calcium levels in three ways:

1. It acts on bones to trigger calcium release.
2. It acts on kidneys to increase the amount of calcium reabsorbed after glomerular filtration so that less calcium is passed in the urine.
3. It acts on kidneys to increase the activation of vitamin D (see below).
   The release of PTH is dependent on having sufficient circulating magnesium.

Calcitriol is the activated form of vitamin D, and is most helpfully viewed as a hormone rather than a nutrient. Ingested vitamin D, and vita-min D made in the skin by the action of ultraviolet light on a precursor compound, undergoes a two-stage activation process (one step in the liver, one in the kidneys) to form calcitriol. Calcitriol has three main actions:

1. It increases calcium absorption from the gut.
2. It acts on kidneys to increase the amount of calcium reabsorbed after glomerular filtration so that less calcium is passed in the urine.

25

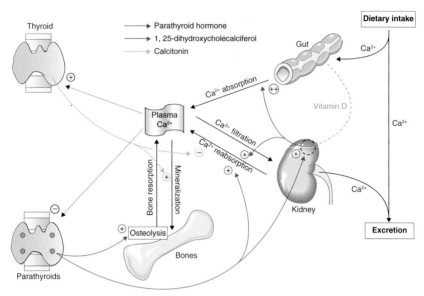

Fig. 4.1 *Homeostatic control mechanisms for calcium (Reproduced with permission from Ward JPT, Linden RWA: Psychology at a Glance (3rd edition), Wiley–Blackwell, 2013.)*

3. It increases calcification of bone.

Calcitonin is another hormone that is involved in calcium homeostasis, but it is less clinically relevant.

When it comes to thinking about causes of hypo- and hypercalcaemia, it is helpful to consider conditions that can affect the body's stores of calcium (e.g., bone cancer causes calcium to be released from bone) and the various hormone systems that should be operating to maintain calcium levels inside a normal range. Normally, in hypocalcaemia, PTH and calcitriol should act to raise calcium levels. In hypercalcaemia, PTH release should cease.

Hypocalcaemia

Contamination of a sample with EDTA can cause a falsely low level of calcium (see Chapter 2).

Common causes are listed in Table 4.1. Useful tests for investigating further include PTH, vitamin D, urea and electrolyte profile, and magnesium.

Hypercalcaemia

Common causes are listed in Table 4.2. Useful tests for investigating further include PTH, vitamin D, urea and electrolyte profile, thyroid function

Cause	Notes
Hypoparathyroidism	PTH is not released appropriately
Vitamin D deficiency (low sunlight exposure or limited diet)	Calcitriol is not produced in adequate quantities
Renal failure	Vitamin D is not activated to calcitriol
Hypomagnesaemia	PTH is not released appropriately

Table 4.1 *Common causes of hypocalcaemia*

Cause	Notes
Malignant cancer, especially when involving bone	Cytokines and other factors released from cancer cells cause calcium release from bone
Primary hyperparathyroidism	Excessive PTH secretion from a (usually) benign parathyroid tumour
Tertiary hyperparathyroidism	Excessive PTH secretion in patients with renal failure who have hypocalcaemia (secondary hyperparathyroidism) can eventually end up with excessive, autonomous secretion of PTH (tertiary hyperparathyroidism)
Hypervitaminosis D	Increased calcitriol production due to excessive consumption of vitamin D
Hyperthyroidism	Excessive bone turnover
Thiazide diuretic treatment	Reduced urinary calcium excretion
Granulomatous disease (sarcoidosis, tuberculosis)	Excessive activation of vitamin D inside granulomata
Familial hypocalciuric hypercalcaemia	A genetic condition where the body interprets a higher-than-normal calcium level as normal due to a faulty calcium sensor

Table 4.2 *Common causes of hypercalcaemia*

tests and urinary calcium excretion. Remember that in hypercalcaemia, the parathyroid glands should stop producing PTH. The finding of a normal or elevated PTH level in the setting of hypercalcaemia should raise suspicions of hyperparathyroidism.

The concept of 'adjusted calcium'

Over one-third of circulating calcium is bound to protein, mostly albumin. Around half circulates as a free ion. If albumin concentrations significantly differ from normal, total calcium results may not give a true reflection of active calcium. It is therefore commonplace to adjust calcium results for albumin.

If albumin is less than 40 g/L, adjusted calcium = measured calcium + 0.02 × (40 − albumin).

If albumin is more than 45 g/L, adjusted calcium = measured calcium − 0.02 × (albumin − 45).

These calculations are generally performed automatically by the laboratory computer system. Pay attention to the adjusted calcium result when making management decisions about a patient.

PHOSPHATE

It may be helpful to think of phosphate problems in a similar way to potassium, as shown in Fig. 4.2. Like potassium, most phosphate is found inside cells rather than in the blood.

Knowledge of key hormone actions will also help in your understanding of phosphate problems. In addition to its effects on calcium, PTH acts on bone and kidneys to lower phosphate. Calcitriol increases phosphate absorption from the gut. In addition, a series of hormones called phosphatonins (e.g., fibroblast growth factor 23) increase phosphate excretion in the urine.

Hypophosphataemia

A common cause for hypophosphataemia is hyperventilation in an anxious person undergoing a blood test. If an isolated fall in phosphate is observed in an otherwise well patient, often repeating the test when the patient is more settled will show a normalised phosphate concentration. Other causes are listed in Table 4.3.

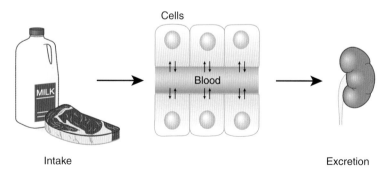

Fig. 4.2 *A simple model of a factory which can assist in understanding some electrolyte abnormalities*

Too little in	Malnutrition
	Vitamin D deficiency
Shift from blood	Hyperventilation (causing alkalosis)
into cells	Carbohydrate infusion
	Treatment of diabetic ketoacidosis
	Re-feeding syndrome
Too much out	Hyperparathyroidism
	Renal tubular leak
	Hypophosphataemic rickets

Table 4.3   *Common causes of hypophosphataemia*

Hyperphosphataemia

Causes are listed in Table 4.4.

Cause	Notes
Renal failure	Reduced phosphate excretion
Rhabdomyolysis	Phosphate is released from damaged cells
Tumour lysis syndrome	Phosphate is released from damaged cells

Table 4.4   *Common causes of hyperphosphataemia*

ALBUMIN

See Chapter 8.

ALKALINE PHOSPHATASE (ALP)

Contamination of a sample with EDTA can cause a falsely low level of ALP (see Chapter 2).

ALP can originate from several parts of the body but predominantly comes from bone or liver/biliary tissue, other sources being intestinal and placental. It is possible to test for ALP isoforms (in particular the 'bone-specific ALP' can often be specifically analysed), which can be helpful in determining the origin of ALP, but for pragmatic purposes, one should inspect a concomitant gamma glutamyl transpeptidase (GGT) result (see Chapter 5) – commonly analysed as part of a liver enzymes panel. If both ALP and GGT are raised, it is likely that the high ALP is of liver/biliary origin. If only ALP is raised, it has likely come from bone. Causes of low and high ALP are shown in Tables 4.5 and 4.6, respectively.

29

Sample contamination with EDTA
Rarely – hypophosphatasia

Table 4.5 *Causes of low ALP*

Bone source (GGT usually normal)
Osteomalacia
Rickets
Paget's disease of bone
Hyperparathyroidism
Cancer affecting bone
Fracture
Liver/biliary source (GGT usually raised)
Cholestasis – see Chapter 5
Intestinal source
Inflammatory bowel disease
Placental source
Late pregnancy

Table 4.6 *Common causes of high ALP*

PUTTING IT ALL TOGETHER

Often a unifying diagnosis can be made with some certainty when component parts of a bone profile are considered together. Common conditions and characteristic findings are listed in Table 4.7.

	Adjusted calcium	Phosphate	ALP	PTH
Primary hyperparathyroidism	↑	↓	↑ or normal	↑
Severe vitamin D deficiency (osteomalacia)	↓	↓	↑	↑
Paget's disease of bone	Normal	Normal	↑	Normal
Bone metastases	↑	↑ or normal	↑ or normal	↓
Hypoparathyroidism	↓	↑	Normal	↓ or normal

Note that when the disorder is one primarily affecting PTH (i.e. hyper- or hypoparathyroidism), calcium and phosphate shift in opposite directions. Vitamin D deficiency causes both to fall.

Table 4.7 *Patterns of test results in common bone diseases*

The liver profile

BILIRUBIN

Bilirubin is largely derived from the breakdown of haem, a key constituent of haemoglobin. Normally, bilirubin is transported to the liver and acted on by enzymes which conjugate it with glucuronic acid, a process which renders the bilirubin water soluble. It is then excreted in bile, and acted on by bacteria in the intestines, forming urobilinogen and then stercobilin. Some urobilinogen is reabsorbed and may be excreted in the urine. Too much circulating bilirubin causes a yellowish discoloration of the skin and sclera and has several causes. Differentiating between these causes is key when interpreting high bilirubin results, and Fig. 5.1 might be helpful in this regard.

High bilirubin may result from any of the processes shown in Table 5.1.

Although it would be helpful to be able to measure conjugated and unconjugated bilirubin separately, these substances are not measured in most laboratories. Instead, 'direct' and 'indirect' bilirubin are often reported, and this difference in terminology can be a cause for confusion. These terms are derived from the fact that the chemical reactions utilised in the laboratory occur readily (or directly) with some forms of bilirubin but not (and hence 'indirectly') with others. For most purposes, it is convenient to consider direct haemoglobin as conjugated and indirect haemoglobin as unconjugated, but readers should realise that this is an oversimplification.

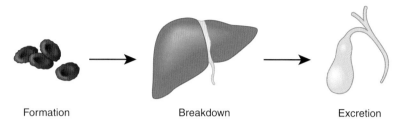

Formation   Breakdown   Excretion

Fig. 5.1 *Bilirubin problems often arise from issues at one of three possible steps*

Mechanism	Common causes	Notes
Excessive bilirubin formation (pre-hepatic)	Haemolysis (abnormal red blood cell breakdown)	Bilirubin generation exceeds capacity of liver to conjugate
Insufficient bilirubin breakdown (hepatic)	Liver disease, e.g., hepatitis, cirrhosis Abnormal conjugating enzymes, e.g., Gilbert's syndrome Effects of drugs on the liver, e.g., rifampicin	Bilirubin is not processed normally by the liver either because of liver damage or abnormal liver enzyme activity
Insufficient bilirubin excretion (post-hepatic)	Blockage to the biliary system, e.g., gallstones Effects of drugs on bile excretion	Biliary production is normal, but it cannot be excreted as normal

Table 5.1 *Mechanisms underlying hyperbilirubinaemia*

Haemolytic anaemia and Gilbert's syndrome

These two conditions often cause confusion when interpreting an elevated bilirubin result, especially when 'liver enzymes' are normal. Haemolysis in this setting describes the abnormal breakdown of red blood cells inside the body (cf. haemolysis outside the body, see Chapter 2). When red cells are destroyed, the bilirubin concentration will rise due to haemoglobin breakdown, but the circulating concentration of other substances will also be altered as follows:

- anaemia (low haemoglobin concentration)
- high reticulocyte count (bone marrow produces immature red blood cells in response)

- increased amounts of circulating enzymes normally found in red cells, e.g., lactate dehydrogenase and aspartate aminotransferase
- low concentrations of haptoglobin (a protein that mops up haemoglobin).

Gilbert's syndrome is a very common phenomenon that is of little clinical relevance (other than causing concern over an abnormal bilirubin result!). The condition is the result of a person conjugating bilirubin less readily than normal. Typical features include a raised bilirubin concentration (usually <100 μmol/L, mainly unconjugated in nature, that rises with illness and fasting) and normal 'liver enzymes'. Haemolysis should generally be excluded by checking the tests mentioned above before making this provisional diagnosis. Genetic confirmation is possible, but often not performed.

'LIVER ENZYMES'

Liver disease can remain silent until it is quite advanced. Often, the first sign of a liver problem is the detection of an abnormality on a panel of 'liver enzymes' checked as part of a general health screening exercise. Studying the pattern of abnormalities on the four enzymes commonly tested can be helpful in deciding what might be wrong with the patient.

Alanine aminotransferase (ALT) and aspartate aminotransferase (AST)

ALT and AST are key enzymes in hepatocytes, and when these cells are damaged, the enzymes spill out into the bloodstream where they are detected in higher than normal quantities. Both enzymes are also found in tissues outside the liver, such as skeletal muscle and heart. Damage to any of these tissues will result in high circulating levels of ALT and AST, and it can be difficult to know which organ system is under stress. The following steps might help:

- Ask the patient! Sore muscles or cardiac-sounding chest pain might be present to point you in the right direction.
- If you suspect damage to another tissue, there may be a more specific test that can be requested, e.g., troponin for myocardial damage or creatine kinase for skeletal muscle.
- Bear in mind that ALT is more specific for liver disease than is AST.

Gamma glutamyl transpeptidase (GGT)

Elevated levels of GGT usually indicate a degree of 'irritation' of liver cells. GGT rises in individuals who regularly consume alcohol, but elevations in GGT are not sufficiently sensitive or specific to allow this test to be used to identify individuals who have recently been drinking. GGT also tends to rise with any cause of cholestasis and in many causes of hepatitis.

Alkaline phosphatase (ALP)

See Chapter 4 for a general overview of ALP. When ALP and GGT are both raised, the ALP is likely to be of liver/biliary origin.

Putting it all together

When assessing ALT, AST, GGT and ALP results, look for patterns as well as abnormalities in the individual test results. In many liver/biliary diseases, levels of all four enzymes will be raised, but often a clear pattern is present as shown in Fig. 5.2. Common causes of deranged 'liver enzymes' are listed in Table 5.2.

SCREENING FOR THE CAUSE OF LIVER DISEASE

Because of the non-diagnostic nature of the liver tests mentioned thus far, it is often necessary to undertake a screening exercise to ascertain the underlying cause of liver disease in a patient (see Table 5.3). Often the cause will be apparent from the clinical presentation, but frequently this is not the case. In some circumstances a liver biopsy will be required for a definitive diagnosis. Imaging of the liver is also often undertaken, and all results taken together to form a diagnosis.

OTHER TESTS IN LIVER DISEASE

Albumin — see Chapter 8. The liver produces albumin, so the level can fall in liver failure.

Alpha-feto protein — see Chapter 11. This is a tumour marker that is used in the surveillance of hepatocellular carcinoma.

HEPATITIC PICTURE	CHOLESTATIC PICTURE
ALT ↑ ↑	ALP ↑ ↑
AST ↑ ↑	GGT ↑ ↑
ALP ↑	ALT ↑
GGT ↑	AST ↑

Fig. 5.2 *Characteristic patterns of liver enzyme abnormalities*

Hepatitic picture, i.e. inflamed liver cells	Viral infection Alcohol Fatty liver disease Autoimmune hepatitis Paracetamol poisoning Other drugs or toxins Wilson disease Liver cancer Right heart failure Primary biliary cirrhosis
Cholestatic picture, i.e. impairment of bile formation or blockage to bile flow	Gallstones Bile duct stricture Cholangiocarcinoma Cancer of the head of pancreas Fatty liver disease Lymphadenopathy around bile duct Ampullary carcinoma Primary sclerosing cholangitis Various drugs Liver cancer

Table 5.2 *Common causes of deranged 'liver enzymes'*

Disease or toxin	Useful additional blood tests	Notes
Alcohol	Mean cell volume (MCV) – see Chapter 15 Carbohydrate-deficient transferrin (CDT) IgA	People who consume alcohol frequently tend to have – high GGT – high MCV – high CDT – high IgA But all of these are non-specific and not suitable for screening purposes
Alpha-1 antitrypsin deficiency	Alpha-1 antitrypsin level and phenotype	See Chapter 8
Autoimmune hepatitis	IgG Anti-nuclear antibody Anti-smooth muscle antibody Anti-liver/kidney microsomal antibody Many other antibodies may be associated	High IgG is common

continued

Disease or toxin	Useful additional blood tests	Notes
Coeliac disease	Anti-endomysial antibody IgA anti-tissue transglutaminase antibody Deamidated anti-gliadin antibody	Problems may arise in patients with IgA deficiency. IgG antibodies may be measured in these individuals
Haemochromatosis	Iron Ferritin Transferrin Transferrin saturation Genetic testing	Typically expect – high ferritin – high transferrin saturation e.g., >50% in males and >40% in females See Chapter 12 Common HFE gene mutations include C282Y and H63D
Paracetamol poisoning	Paracetamol level at least 4 hours post-ingestion – see Chapter 13	Low levels (or none) may be detected if checked late after ingestion
Primary biliary cirrhosis	IgM Anti-mitochondrial antibody (AMA) Anti-nuclear antibody (PBC-specific subtypes) Genetic testing	High IgM is typical
Viral hepatitis	Antigen testing, RNA/DNA testing, antibody testing for viruses that can cause hepatitis	Common viruses are hepatitis A/B/C/E, Epstein Barr virus and Cytomegalovirus
Wilson disease	Caeruloplasmin Urinary copper Genetics	Typically expect – low caeruloplasmin High urinary copper

Table 5.3 *Diseases causing liver dysfunction*

Ammonia — see Chapter 14. The liver is involved in protein metabolism; thus elevated ammonia levels can occur in liver failure.

Coagulation screen — see Chapter 16. The liver produces clotting factors; therefore coagulopathy is common in liver failure.

Tests for fibrosis — several tests may be combined in an attempt to ascertain if a patient has developed liver fibrosis. One such system is the Enhanced Liver Fibrosis (ELF) score that utilises results from three special tests: tissue inhibitor of metalloproteinases 1, amino-terminal propeptide of type III procollagen and hyaluronic acid.

Blood gas analysis and pH

SAMPLE REQUIREMENTS

In contrast to most other blood tests, gas analysis and pH measurement is usually performed using whole blood. A blood sample is typically withdrawn into a specially designed syringe that comes with a small amount of heparin inside the chamber to stop clotting. It is important that any air remaining in the syringe is expelled after sample collection, otherwise gas exchange will occur between this air and the collected blood, and results will be affected. Samples are generally analysed using a POCT analyser. It is important to know whether blood has been sampled from an artery or vein when considering oxygen results, as much lower levels of oxygen would be expected from a vein.

CORE COMPONENTS OF THE TEST PANEL

POCT analysers are often set up to measure the concentrations of a large number of substances in the sample, e.g., electrolytes, glucose and lactate. Additionally, they often report 'calculated indices' which are results that the machine calculates after analysis is complete. Of particular importance is the fact that measures of bicarbonate from POCT analysers are usually calculated. You may come across the term 'standard bicarbonate'. This is a further calculated index that attempts to provide information on what the bicarbonate concentration would be if the respiratory components of the disorder were eliminated. 'Base excess' is another calculated index which

	What it actually means	Simple meaning
pH	$-\log_{10}$ [H⁺] (where [H⁺] is the concentration of hydrogen ions (measured in mol/L)	Acidity
P_aO_2	Partial pressure of oxygen	Oxygen content
P_aCO_2	Partial pressure of carbon dioxide	Carbon dioxide content
Bicarbonate	Concentration of bicarbonate	Bicarbonate content

Table 6.1 *The major parts of a blood gas report*

will be elevated in the setting of metabolic alkalosis and reduced in metabolic acidosis. In most cases, the majority of information from a blood gas analysis can be gleaned by assessing the information in Table 6.1.

ACID-BASE STATUS

Interpretation of pH, P_aCO_2 and bicarbonate results in combination is essential when assessing a patient's acid-base status. The pH is normally tightly regulated between 7.35 and 7.45. 'Acidaemia' refers to a pH below this range and 'alkalaemia' to a pH above this range. Sometimes, hydrogen ion concentration ([H⁺]) may be provided in lieu of pH, but both are related, since pH = $-\log_{10}$ [H⁺] (where [H⁺] is in mol/L). Note the minus sign before the 'log' operator: as a solution becomes more acidic, the H⁺ rises but the pH falls.

Biological systems do not like abnormal pH! The human body has two mechanisms that can be used to keep pH on track. First, buffers are present in blood; the key buffer for understanding most acid-base problems is bicarbonate. Healthy kidneys can generate bicarbonate and reclaim any that has filtered through the glomeruli. Second, the body can alter the amount of carbon dioxide exhaled during ventilation. The body will use these systems to try to normalise pH once it deviates away from normality.

A low bicarbonate concentration either means that the bicarbonate is being used up buffering excess hydrogen ions, or that it is being lost from the gastrointestinal tract or in the urine, or that the kidneys are failing to generate sufficient bicarbonate. A low bicarbonate concentration is the key finding in metabolic acidosis. An increased bicarbonate concentration can occur when acidic fluid is lost from the body and is a feature of metabolic alkalosis.

Think of carbon dioxide as an acidic gas (you may recall from your chemistry studies that carbonic acid is formed when carbon dioxide

Acidosis		Alkalosis	
Metabolic	Large number of causes. **Calculate anion gap to assist**. See below for details.	Metabolic	Saline responsive: **vomiting, diarrhoea, diuretics, extracellular volume contraction** Not saline responsive: Mineralocorticoid excess, e.g., Cushing's syndrome, hyperaldosteronism, hypokalaemia
Respiratory	**Respiratory disease,** e.g., chronic obstructive pulmonary disorder **Depressed respiratory drive** due to drugs or central nervous system pathology **Mechanical problem with ventilation,** e.g., chest wall injury	Respiratory	**Hyperventilation,** e.g., due to hypoxia (which has a large number of causes), stimulation of the respiratory centre (e.g., salicylate poisoning, hyperammonaemia) or psychological

Table 6.2 *Common causes of acid-base abnormalities*

dissolves in water). By increasing carbon dioxide excretion, the lungs can effectively clear acid from the body. If the body has an ongoing disease process generating a metabolic acidosis, the respiratory rate should increase and the P_aCO_2 should fall in an attempt to correct the pH back towards normality. A low P_aCO_2 thus indicates a respiratory alkalosis. In many respiratory diseases and in conditions where respiratory function is compromised, P_aCO_2 can rise and result in respiratory acidosis.

Once you have established the pH and whether there is a metabolic/respiratory acidosis/alkalosis, you should move on to work out the cause by considering the patient's details and arranging further investigations as necessary. Common causes are shown in Table 6.2.

Anion gap

Metabolic acidosis is the commonest acid-base problem in acutely unwell patients, and there are a large number of potential causes. To assist in finding the likely cause, the **anion gap** should be calculated. The number of positive charges (cations) present in blood equals the number of negative charges (anions). If it were feasible to measure all charged substances in blood, it could be shown that the sum of the positively charged particles is exactly balanced by the number of those substances carrying negative charges. It is routine practice to measure only four charged particles: sodium, potassium, chloride and bicarbonate ions. As discussed earlier, total CO_2 on a urea and electrolyte profile may be considered as a convenient surrogate measure of bicarbonate and can be used in the calculation of the anion gap. When the number of cations (sodium and potassium) are added, one will always find that they outnumber the anions (chloride and bicarbonate). This difference is the anion gap. An anion gap may be low, normal or high, and can be conveniently calculated as follows:

Anion Gap = (Sodium + Potassium) – (Chloride + Bicarbonate)
(where all concentrations are in mmol/L)
Potassium is often ignored, making the calculation simpler:
Anion Gap = (Sodium) – (Chloride + Bicarbonate)

The reference interval (normal range) for anion gap varies from laboratory to laboratory, and is inherently imprecise because of the number of measurements required for its calculation. An anion gap greater than 20 mmol/L is always considered to be abnormally elevated and a gap of less than 10 mmol/L abnormally low. The author's approach is to actively seek out causes of a high anion gap in patients with gaps exceeding 14 mmol/L (or 18 mmol/L if potassium is included in the equation above). Anion gaps below the reference interval are uncommon. Causes include laboratory error and low protein states.

Once the anion gap has been calculated, decide whether it is high, normal or low, and then try to establish the cause by considering the patient's details and arranging further investigations as necessary. High anion gap metabolic acidosis causes can be recalled using the mnemonic 'GOLD MARK', but the three commonest causes (shown in bold in the Table 6.3) should always be considered first.

Metabolic Acidosis	
High anion gap	**Normal anion gap**
Glycols (e.g., ethylene glycol poisoning)	**Gastrointestinal bicarbonate loss,** e.g.,
Oxoproline excess	high-output ileostomy, diarrhoea
L-lactic acidosis	Renal bicarbonate loss, e.g., renal tubule
D-lactic acidosis	damage, type 2 renal tubular acidosis
Methanol	Types 1 and 4 renal tubular acidosis
Aspirin poisoning	
Renal failure	
Ketoacidosis	

Table 6.3 *Common causes of metabolic acidosis*

Glycols and methanol can be tested for on special arrangement with the laboratory (see Chapter 13). Ethylene glycol (antifreeze) is uncommonly taken in overdose and is particularly toxic. Oxoproline (also known as pyroglutamic acid) toxicity occurs most often in older, malnourished patients who have chronic paracetamol exposure or who have been on certain antibiotics. It can be detected in urine during an organic acid screen. L-lactic acid is the commonly found form of lactate, often seen in patients with organ hypoperfusion. D-lactic acid can be found in patients with abnormalities of the gut (see Chapter 14). Aspirin poisoning can be detected on a salicylate test (see Chapter 13). Renal failure will be apparent on a urea and electrolyte profile (see Chapter 3). Ketoacidosis can be diagnosed after a ketone estimation (see Chapter 9).

PARTIAL PRESSURE OF OXYGEN (P_aO_2)

It is imperative that the inspired oxygen concentration is known before interpreting a P_aO_2 result. If a patient is breathing high-flow oxygen, their P_aO_2 should be much higher than the reference range, which is designed for interpreting results from patients breathing 21% oxygen.

If a person is breathing 'room air' with an inspired oxygen concentration (FiO_2) of 21% at sea level, the standard reference range for P_aO_2 will apply. If the patient is breathing supplemental oxygen or is at high altitude, a variety of factors will determine the expected P_aO_2. One should first estimate the partial pressure of oxygen in the alveoli (P_AO_2 – note uppercase 'A') as follows:

$$P_AO_2 = FiO_2 (P_b\text{-}P_{H2O}) - P_aCO_2/RQ$$

where P_b denotes barometric pressure, P_{H2O} denotes partial pressure of water, and RQ denotes 'respiratory quotient' which is a factor dependent on metabolic rate.

The alveolar-arterial (A-a) gradient can then be calculated as P_AO_2–P_aO_2. The expected A-a gradient varies by age and can be approximated using the following equation: A-a gradient = (Age + 10)/4. An abnormally high A-a gradient indicates pathology in the lungs.

A useful rule of thumb which works quite well in practice is to subtract 10 from the FiO_2 (when given in percentage terms) to estimate the expected P_aO_2 in kPa. Thus a P_aO_2 of 11 kPa would be expected for someone breathing 21% oxygen, but would be extremely abnormal for a ventilated patient on 100% oxygen.

PARTIAL PRESSURE OF CARBON DIOXIDE (P_aCO_2)

As mentioned under the assessment of acid-base status, the speed and effectiveness of ventilation determines the P_aCO_2. Low results are found

Respiratory failure	P_aO_2	P_aCO_2
Type 1	<8 kPa	Normal or low
Type 2	<8 kPa	High

Table 6.4 *Types of respiratory failure*

in hyperventilatory states and result in a respiratory alkalosis. High levels are seen with hypoventilation and cause respiratory acidosis. Refer to Table 6.2 for common causes.

With the P_aO_2 and P_aCO_2 results in hand, one can assess if a patient has 'respiratory failure' and classify its type (see Table 6.4).

CARBOXYHAEMOGLOBIN

The carboxyhaemoglobin concentration will be markedly raised in cases of carbon monoxide poisoning and slightly elevated in smokers.

Endocrine testing

Endocrine diseases result from an excess or a deficiency in one or more hormones. Knowledge of how the key hormone systems are regulated in health will make interpretation of endocrine blood tests more straightforward. For many hormones, a three-stage control system is in operation. To conceptualise this, consider a factory worker with two tiers of managers (Fig. 7.1).

There is communication between the three people in this system, with each communicating to the tier above and below about the amount of work being done. For the hypothalamic-pituitary axis, a similar system is present, although sometimes the situation is a little more complex, e.g., with the worker talking back to the manager directly, or more than one manager controlling a worker. These processes are normally called negative feedback loops, and are the body's way of ensuring that 'just enough' hormone is produced.

When assessing any set of endocrine results, the approach shown in Fig. 7.2 should be useful.

GLANDS CONTROLLED BY THE ANTERIOR PITUITARY

Convention dictates that if the end-gland is faulty, the problem is a 'primary' one, whereas if the pituitary is faulty, the problem is a secondary one. A full assessment of anterior pituitary function involves checking each hormone axis controlled by it.

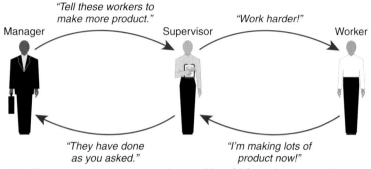

Fig. 7.1 The 'manager, supervisor, worker' model useful for understanding the hypothalamic-pituitary axis

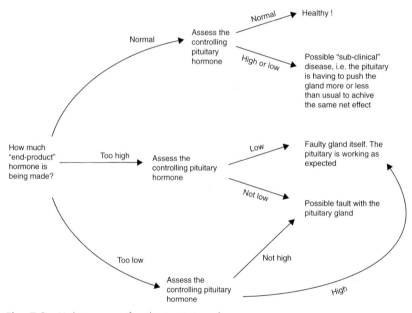

Fig. 7.2 Making sense of endocrine test results

Thyroid

The two main problems to be diagnosed on blood testing are hypo- and hyperthyroidism. Establishment of the cause of the problem should be attempted next.

Two tests are generally reported in thyroid function panels: free thyroxine and thyroid-stimulating hormone (TSH). Common patterns of results are shown in Table 7.1. Beware of checking thyroid function in a patient who is acutely unwell. Due to the effects of various inflammatory mediators, thyroid function tests can be abnormal in people with a normally heathy thyroid axis. This phenomenon is known as euthyroid sick syndrome or non-thyroidal illness syndrome.

To identify most problems, look at the free thyroxine result first and then decide what the TSH 'should' be doing in that circumstance if the pituitary was working normally. Then look at the TSH result to see what is happening in that particular patient. In a primary thyroid gland problem, tests can then be undertaken to ascertain the cause of the faulty gland. If a pituitary problem is suspected, full pituitary testing should be carried out.

Further blood testing can be performed as required, and other investigations may be necessary. Other important tests include the following:

- Free triiodothyronine (T_3) (formed from thyroxine) — T_3 thyrotoxicosis is possible
- Autoantibodies, e.g., anti-thyroid peroxidase (TPO) (found in Hashimoto's thyroiditis and Graves' disease), thyroglobulin antibody (found in Hashimoto's thyroiditis), TSH-receptor antibody (found in Graves' disease)
- Evidence of inflammation, e.g., ESR — in thyroiditis

	Free thyroxine	TSH
Primary hyperthyroidism	↑	↓
Secondary hyperthyroidism*	↑	Normal or ↑
Primary hypothyroidism	↓	↑
Secondary hypothyroidism	↓	Normal or ↓
Subclinical hyperthyroidism**	Normal	↓
Subclinical hypothyroidism	Normal	↑

*Uncommonly, this pattern can be seen due to interference with the laboratory assay. Repeating the testing on a different laboratory platform will identify this. The rare syndrome of thyroid hormone resistance will also produce results like this.

**Need to check free triiodothyronine (T_3, see below) in case the patient has T_3 thyrotoxicosis.

Table 7.1 Common patterns of thyroid hormone results

Adrenals

The two main problems to be diagnosed are hypo- and hyperadrenalism. Establishment of the cause of the problem should be attempted next. Initial blood testing should be guided by the clinical picture. Straightforward testing of cortisol can be performed, but cortisol exhibits a marked diurnal variation in release, so a one-off cortisol level is usually not particularly helpful. The exception to this rule is a very low cortisol concentration shortly after waking which is suggestive of hypoadrenalism, since cortisol levels should be fairly high at this time of the day.

Hypoadrenalism

The commonest first-line test for hypoadrenalism is the short Synacthen test. Synacthen is SYNthetic adrenocorticotrophic hormone (ACTH) injected into the patient in an attempt to stimulate the adrenal cortex to produce cortisol. If normally functioning, the cortisol level should rise over a defined decision level after 30 minutes. If the 30-minute cortisol level is lower than expected, proceed to look at a 9 a.m. ACTH level to distinguish primary from secondary hypoadrenalism. Other techniques of assessing adrenal function may be advised by an endocrinologist. Once primary or secondary hypoadrenalism is confirmed, proceed to investigate for a cause.

You might wonder why the response to Synacthen is abnormal in most cases of secondary hypoadrenalism as logic dictates that the adrenal gland should be healthy and respond normally to stimulation. However, the reason for this is that the adrenal gland tends to atrophy if it is not being stimulated over a period of time. The same response is often seen in patients who have been on long-term corticosteroid treatment.

Hyperadrenalism

Hyperadrenalism produces the features of Cushing's syndrome. The initial test for this is usually a 24-hour urine collection for free cortisol, an elevated level being grounds for further investigation. A common second-line investigation is a dexamethasone suppression test. There are several variants of this, but in the relatively straightforward overnight suppression test, patients are given dexamethasone at night before having cortisol checked at 9 a.m. In health, the adrenal glands detect the dexamethasone and switch off cortisol production, so a low level should be obtained. In hyperadrenalism, cortisol production continues and an elevated level is expected. Once confirmed, an endocrinologist can investigate for a cause. In hyperadrenalism secondary to a pituitary tumour, cortisol production will suppress after the administration of several large doses of dexamethasone (the 'high-dose dexamethasone suppression test') – cortisol production will continue at a high level in other causes. Sometimes endocrinologists will perform a corticotrophin-releasing hormone test. Administration of this hormone will result in a significant rise in ACTH and cortisol in patients with a pituitary cause. Once primary or secondary hyperadrenalism is confirmed, proceed to investigate for a cause.

Primary hyperaldosteronism

A primary adrenal gland problem is the key diagnosis of exclusion in cases of hyperaldosteronism. The first-line investigation involves measuring aldosterone and renin, and then calculating their ratio. If this 'aldosterone:renin' ratio is abnormal (in keeping with a high aldosterone and relatively low renin), then further confirmatory testing can be performed. A common second-line investigation is a saline suppression test. In health, the intravenous infusion of saline will result in a marked reduction in aldosterone secretion. Once confirmed, further specialist testing can be performed to define the cause of the primary hyperaldosteronism.

Congenital adrenal hyperplasia (CAH)

Fig. 7.3 shows a simplified version of the metabolic pathway for the synthesis of cortisol. The commonest enzyme defect that results in CAH is 21-hydroxylase deficiency. The key test for diagnosing CAH is measurement of 17-hydroxyprogesterone (17-OHP), which will be elevated in patients with this condition. In infants, it is important to delay testing of 17-OHP for at least 2 days after birth to ensure that it is not maternal hormone that is being detected.

Phaeochromocytoma and paraganglioma

Phaeochromocytoma is the term used to describe a tumour of the adrenal medulla that secretes excessive quantities of catecholamines. Paragangliomas are similar tumours arising from sympathetic paravertebral ganglia. Catecholamines produced in such tissues are acted on by an enzyme (catecholamine O-methyltransferase) that converts them into normetadrenaline and metadrenaline, which are collectively known as metanephrines. Measurement of the concentration of metanephrines in the blood is a good initial screening test for these disorders. Once suspected, specialised testing to locate and characterise the tumours further can be undertaken.

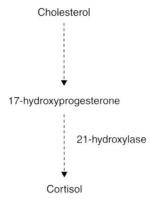

Fig. 7.3 *A simplified version of the cortisol synthetic pathway*

Gonads

Males

The main problem to be diagnosed on blood testing is hypogonadism. The hallmark of male hypogonadism is low testosterone. Establishment of the cause of the problem should be attempted next. If testosterone is low, look at the luteinising hormone (LH) and follicle-stimulating hormone (FSH) levels to differentiate between a testicular problem (primary hypogonadism, when LH and FSH will be high) and a pituitary problem (when they will not be high). Further investigations can then be arranged to probe deeper. Most circulating testosterone is bound to protein (mainly sex hormone binding globulin (SHBG) and albumin), but it is only 'free' hormone that is metabolically active. In some cases, SHBG concentrations can be altered, thus affecting the amount of free hormone. There are calculating tools available for calculating the amount of free testosterone from commonly reported laboratory values.

Females

Interpreting gonadal hormones in pre-menopausal adult females is a more complex task than that in males, because of the cyclical variation. When interpreting such results, one should be cognisant of which part of the menstrual cycle the patient is in at the time of blood sampling. Rather than working through results using first principles, it is often easier to look for familiar patterns in results. In practice, testing is usually performed in a particular clinical context (e.g., infertility or amenorrhoea), and the interpretation of results is more meaningful when likely pathologies are borne in mind.

Ovarian failure. In failure of the ovaries (one common cause of which is menopause), oestradiol levels will be low while LH and FSH levels will be high (i.e. comparable situation to primary hypogonadism in males). Secondary ovarian failure is a much less common situation, but will result in low oestradiol with normal or low LH and FSH.

Polycystic ovarian syndrome. Various biochemical abnormalities can be present in this condition, but the key finding is evidence of hyperandrogenism. Testosterone and 'free androgen index' are commonly reported; other androgens can be tested if required. When SHBG concentrations are known, free testosterone can be calculated, as above. Beware of the woman with very high androgen levels who may have an androgen-secreting tumour.

Ovulatory failure. A low progesterone on day 21 of the menstrual cycle is evidence of failure to ovulate that can then be investigated further (e.g., with pituitary investigations).

Pregnancy. Human chorionic gonadotrophin (hCG) is produced in the placenta, and testing for it is the basis of most pregnancy tests. In early pregnancy, hCG levels increase rapidly. In ectopic pregnancies, hCG rises but at a slower rate.

Growth hormone (GH)

The main problem to be diagnosed on blood testing in adults is acromegaly, caused by GH excess. GH acts on the liver causing the release of insulin-like growth factor 1 (IGF-1), and elevated levels of IGF-1 are the hallmark of acromegaly. Confirmation of the diagnosis can be done by checking GH levels 2 hours after the administration of 75 g of glucose by mouth. In health, GH levels are suppressed in this setting.

Growth hormone deficiency in adults is usually diagnosed after either an insulin tolerance test or a glucagon stimulation test, under the guidance of an endocrinologist. In an insulin tolerance test, the patient is rendered hypoglycaemic (in a carefully monitored setting), and the GH level should rise as part of the body's stress response. For poorly understood reasons, GH should also rise after the administration of glucagon.

Prolactin

Prolactin is involved in lactation, but its measurement is of particular interest in pituitary disease as it tends to rise in many pituitary tumours. This happens because pituitary enlargement impedes blood flow into the gland

Cause	Notes
Macro-prolactin	Normally excluded by a laboratory automatically
Physiological	e.g., breastfeeding, pregnancy
Drugs	e.g., metoclopramide, phenothiazine antipsychotics
Pituitary tumours	
Hypothyroidism	
Chronic kidney disease	
Polycystic ovarian syndrome	

Table 7.2 *Common causes of elevated prolactin*

from the hypothalamus. The hypothalamus normally sends dopamine to the pituitary to switch off prolactin secretion. In the absence of this dopamine signal, prolactin secretion increases.

The concept of macro-enzymes is described in Chapter 8 and is of particular relevance to prolactin. Laboratories routinely check for the presence of macro-prolactin before releasing results. Macro-prolactin is a compound comprising regular prolactin joined to an immunoglobulin molecule. Some people carry macro-prolactin which is of no consequence, so it is important that laboratories can identify this and distinguish it from true hyperprolactinaemia. Common causes of elevated prolactin are listed in Table 7.2.

TESTING POSTERIOR PITUITARY FUNCTION

Oxytocin function is not assessed clinically, meaning that the activity of antidiuretic hormone (ADH) is the only posterior pituitary hormone considered here.

Water deprivation test

This is used to differentiate diabetes insipidus (DI) from primary polydipsia, which can both cause polyuria. In primary polydipsia, patients drink excessively, often for psychological reasons. Thinking a little about the pathophysiology of these conditions can help interpret results from a water deprivation test.

1. Primary polydipsia. The patient drinks excessively. As a result, they appropriately pass large volumes of dilute urine. If they are stopped from drinking, the urine volume decreases and becomes more concentrated.

2. DI. The patient's ADH is not working correctly, either because it is no longer being produced (cranial DI) or because it is not acting correctly on the kidneys (nephrogenic DI). Think of ADH as a cork which plugs the hole in the bottom of a leaky bucket (see Fig. 7.4).

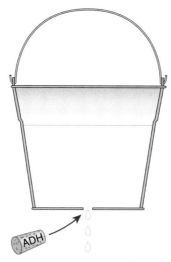

Fig. 7.4 *Anti-diuretic hormone (ADH) stops the loss of water in urine*

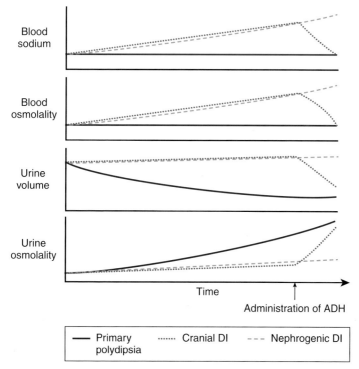

Fig. 7.5 *Characteristic changes during a water deprivation test*

In cranial DI, the corks are not being made. In nephrogenic DI, the corks do not plug the hole. If a patient with DI is stopped from drinking, they will continue to pass large volumes of dilute urine and become very dehydrated (causing blood sodium and osmolality to rise). During the test, they are injected with ADH. If this fixes the problem, they have cranial DI; if not, they have nephrogenic DI.

Fig. 7.5 illustrates the typical variation of measured parameters during a water deprivation test for these various conditions.

Blood proteins and enzymes

OUTLINE

Some proteins and enzymes are considered in other sections of the book, where most appropriate (e.g., liver enzymes are covered in Chapter 5). Other proteins and enzymes are considered here.

AN INTRODUCTION TO BLOOD PROTEINS

A very large number of proteins is present in blood. One way to get a feel for the relative quantities of the various types of protein present is to analyse a sample using electrophoresis. Put simply, electrophoresis is a method of separating out the constituent proteins in a sample to allow an element of analysis to take place. The following diagrams should shed some light on one way that this process is carried out, although currently more sophisticated technologies are often used in many laboratories for the separation stage. First, the sample is processed and loaded onto a support medium and stained. Under appropriate conditions, the different proteins in the sample migrate different distances because of the differing chemical properties. After separation, a trace like that shown in Fig. 8.1 will be obtained.

An optical reader is then used to assess the density of the 'smudges' along this trace. If plotted out, a plot similar to Fig. 8.2 will be obtained.

This characteristic pattern is what is seen in health. Laboratory professionals who interpret such traces have expertise in comparing this standard shape to that of the sample being tested. Characteristic peaks are seen. The largest peak is generally due to the presence of albumin, as it is the protein found in highest concentration in healthy subjects. The alpha-1 (α_1) region comprises various proteins, e.g., α_1-anti-trypsin (note α_1 in the name). The alpha-2 (α_2) region comprises proteins such as α_2-macroglobulin and haptoglobin. Transferrin (and others) is found in the beta (β) region. The gamma (γ) region is made up of immunoglobulins.

In the past, various inferences could be made about a patient's state of health, and cause of ill-health, by studying the shape of the electrophoresis

Fig 8.1 *A typical protein electrophoresis trace*

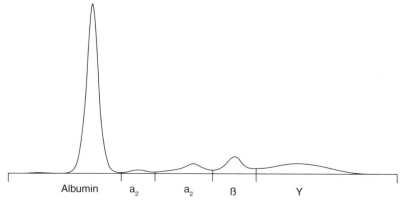

Fig 8.2 *A protein electrophoresis trace from a normal subject*

curve. Nowadays, protein electrophoresis is generally only performed to look for the presence of 'paraprotein'; abnormal protein produced in conditions such as multiple myeloma.

PARAPROTEIN

In inflammatory processes, the gamma region on electrophoresis will often be seen to be elevated, but in a smooth, broad way with no discrete peaks. This is called a 'polyclonal' pattern, as the excessive amounts of protein detected have been produced by a variety of cells. In myeloma and similar conditions, a single line of faulty plasma cells in the bone marrow work in overdrive, such that a single type of immunoglobulin is produced in excess, giving it the term 'monoclonal'. If blood from a patient with such a condition is subjected to electrophoresis, an appearance similar to Fig. 8.3 might be found. You should be able to appreciate the clearly abnormal 'band' toward the right side of the patient's sample.

If the density of the smudges on this sample is then plotted, something like Fig. 8.4 will be obtained.

You can appreciate the large monoclonal peak in the gamma region. Biomedical scientists can then utilise a range of methods to identify the type of protein that is causing the peak. Serum protein electrophoresis reports will thus comprise two main pieces of information:

1. Band type, i.e. the nature of the immunoglobulin causing the peak, IgA, IgM or IgG.
2. Band size, i.e. an estimate of the concentration of the abnormal protein.

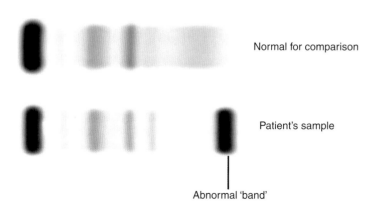

Normal for comparison

Patient's sample

Abnormal 'band'

Fig 8.3 *Normal and abnormal protein electrophoresis traces*

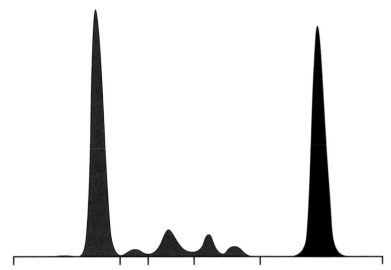

Fig 8.4 *Protein electrophoresis from a subject with significant paraproteinaemia*

Serum free light chains

Immunoglobulins have a general structure as that shown in Fig. 8.5 and have both heavy and light chains.

It is possible to detect circulating free light chains in blood, which are present in addition to the light chains comprising intact immunoglobulin. These will be one of two types, kappa (κ) or lambda (λ), and reports usually detail the concentration of each type present and their ratio. In general inflammatory states, because of polyclonal immunoglobulin production, both types will be elevated. In monoclonal plasma cell disorders, often one type of light chain will be produced in excess, making the ratio abnormal.

Other laboratory findings in multiple myeloma

If multiple myeloma is suspected, several characteristic laboratory abnormalities may be present as shown in Table 8.1.

IMMUNOGLOBULINS

There are several types of immunoglobulins in blood, and it is possible to quantify these. From most to least abundant, the immunoglobulin classes normally present are IgG, IgA, IgM, IgD and IgE. Immunoglobulin levels

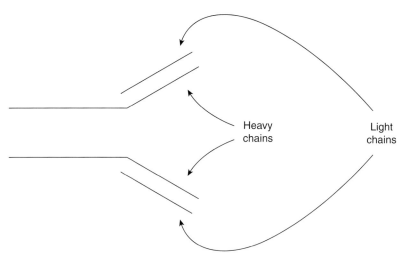

Fig 8.5 *The general structure of immunoglobulins*

Finding	Explanation
Anaemia	Healthy precursor cells in bone marrow overwhelmed with abnormal plasma cells
High ESR	Due to high concentration of circulating proteins
Hypercalcaemia	Lytic lesions in bone release calcium into the circulation
Immunoparesis (low levels of other immunoglobulins)	Healthy precursor cells in bone marrow overwhelmed with abnormal plasma cells
Kidney impairment	Protein, e.g., light chains impair kidney function
Paraprotein	Monoclonal plasma cell production of immunoglobulin

Table 8.1 *Characteristic laboratory abnormalities in multiple myeloma*

change markedly at the time of birth, as circulating maternal Ig is gradually replaced. Low levels of one (e.g., IgA deficiency) or many immunoglobulins may be detected in individuals who may then be at high risk of infection.

High levels of immunoglobulins are detected in many conditions. Specific types of immunoglobulins can point towards a specific disease process, and are often helpful in investigating infectious diseases where antibodies to particular pathogens (types of immunoglobulins) can be measured. Autoantibodies are immunoglobulins which can be helpful in diagnosis. Commonly tested autoantibodies and their linked diseases are shown in Table 8.2. Most autoantibodies are not 100% sensitive or specific for any particular disease.

Autoantibody	Characteristic disease
Anti- double stranded DNA antibody (dsDNA)	SLE
Anti-centromere antibody	CREST syndrome
Anti-cyclic citrullinated peptide antibody (CCP)	Rheumatoid arthritis
Anti-endomysial antibody	Coeliac disease
Anti-glutamate decarboxylase antibody (GAD)	Type 1 diabetes
Anti-glomerular basement membrane antibody (GBM)	Goodpasture's syndrome
Anti-Intrinsic factor antibody	Pernicious anaemia
Anti-Jo-1 antibody	Inflammatory myopathies
Anti-liver-kidney microsomal antibody (LKM)	Autoimmune hepatitis
Anti-mitochondrial antibody (AMA)	Primary biliary cirrhosis
Anti-nuclear antibody (ANA)	Various
Anti-parietal cell antibody	Pernicious anaemia
Anti-ribonucleoprotein antibody (RNP)	Mixed CT disease
Anti-Sjögren syndrome A (Ro) antibody (SS-A)	SLE, Sjögren syndrome
Anti-Sjögren syndrome B (La) antibody (SS-B)	Sjögren syndrome
Anti-Smith antibody (Sm)	SLE
Anti-smooth muscle antibody (SMA)	Autoimmune hepatitis
Anti-thyroglobulin antibody	Hashimoto's thyroiditis
Anti-thyroid peroxidase antibody (TPO)	Hashimoto's / Graves'
Anti-tissue transglutaminase antibody	Coeliac disease
Antri-scleroderma-70 antibody (SCL-70)	Systemic sclerosis
Cytoplasmic-anti-neutrophil cytoplasmic antibody (c-ANCA)	GPA
Perinuclear-anti-neutrophil cytoplasmic antibody (p-ANCA)	EGPA
Rheumatoid factor	Rheumatoid arthritis
Thyroid stimulating hormone receptor antibody	Graves' disease

CT, connective tissue; EGPA, eosinophilic granulomatosis with polyangiitis; GPA, granulomatosis with polyangiitis; SLE, systemic lupus erythematosus

Table 8.2 *Commonly requested autoantibodies*

More generally, characteristic patterns of immunoglobulin elevations can point towards a cause in patients with liver disease (see Chapter 5), and assessment of IgE can be helpful in conditions with an allergic of hypersensitivity aetiology.

TOTAL PROTEIN

Total protein quantifies the amount of protein in a sample but provides no information on what constitutes that protein. The commonest occurring protein in the blood is albumin; most of the rest of circulating proteins are globulins. You should perform the following quick calculation when provided with total protein and albumin results:

Total globulins = total protein – albumin

The finding of a very high globulin concentration should be followed up with testing of immunoglobulins, serum protein electrophoresis and serum free light chains in order to explain this finding. The most important diagnosis to consider is that of multiple myeloma.

ALBUMIN

Albumin measurement is usually undertaken as part of a liver profile (see Chapter 5), as the liver is involved in the synthesis of albumin, or a bone profile, as it is impossible to interpret a calcium measurement without knowing the albumin concentration (see Chapter 4). Common causes of low and high albumin concentrations are listed in Tables 8.3 and 8.4, respectively.

Long-standing malnutrition
Protein-losing enteropathy
Nephrotic syndrome
Acute inflammatory processes
Liver failure

Table 8.3 *Common causes of low albumin*

Dehydration

Table 8.4 *Common cause of high albumin*

α₁-ANTI-TRYPSIN

This is an anti-proteinase enzyme, deficiency of which can cause lung and/or liver disease. The test is often requested when investigating a patient with altered liver enzymes (see Chapter 5), established liver disease or emphysema. Two pieces of information are provided when the test is requested: the amount of α_1-anti-trypsin present and the type.

Amount: expect low levels in deficiency states but beware the patient with an ongoing acute-phase reaction. In this setting, α_1-anti-trypsin rises (like C-reactive protein, see below), and thus a falsely reassuring result might be obtained.

Type: there are lots of variations of α_1-anti-trypsin. Results are expressed in the form 'Piβγ' where 'Pi' refers to protease inhibitor and β and γ refer to the two types of gene that are present in the patient in question. Common types are M, S and Z. A homozygous patient will have both letters the same, e.g., PiZZ; heterozygotes will have different letters, e.g., PiSZ. PiMM is normal. PiSS and PiZZ are most likely to be associated with disease, but heterozygotes may also be affected with the clinical phenotype. You may find it easy to recall the 'Pimm's' drink which is often produced during celebrations to recall that PiMM is normal. You can probably think up your own way of remembering that PiSS and PiZZ are less than ideal!

AMYLASE AND LIPASE

Amylase and lipase are generally checked when acute pancreatitis is suspected. Significantly elevated lipase levels are generally only found in acute pancreatitis.

In contrast, there are many causes of a raised amylase (see Table 8.5). Recall that amylase is produced by the pancreas and by salivary glands. When considering causes for elevated amylase levels, think about diseases which occur 'near' the pancreas and inside salivary glands.

ANGIOTENSIN-CONVERTING ENZYME (ACE)

ACE levels are generally only measured in patients with confirmed or suspected sarcoidosis. In some patients with this condition, ACE is elevated, and tracking changes in ACE with time may be helpful in management. The test is not a sensitive diagnostic tool for this condition, however, as some patients can have sarcoidosis with normal ACE levels.

BONE TURNOVER MARKERS

Bone turnover markers are sometimes requested from specialised metabolic bone clinics and in research studies. Short notes are provided on the most frequently used markers below:

Alkaline phosphatase (ALP) and bone-specific ALP

See Chapter 4.

Acute pancreatitis
Salivary gland calculus
Salivary gland tumour
Other pancreatic disease, e.g., pancreatic cancer, chronic pancreatitis, pseudocyst
Gallbladder disease, e.g., acute cholecystitis
Duodenal disease, e.g., perforated duodenal ulcer
Bowel disease, e.g., bowel obstruction
Intra-abdominal vascular disease, e.g., ruptured aortic aneurysm, mesenteric ischaemia
Uterine disease, e.g., ruptured ectopic pregnancy

Table 8.5 *Causes of high amylase*

Procollagen 1 amino-terminal extension peptide (P1NP)

This is a marker of osteoblast activity and therefore bone formation. A common use for measuring P1NP is in monitoring the therapeutic response to bisphosphonate therapy in patients with osteoporosis. Appropriate treatment should result in a suppression in P1NP levels, but there are several pitfalls, as levels can rise after a fracture and will be higher in patients with renal failure and in children and adolescents who are growing.

C-telopeptide of collagen cross-links (CTX)

This is a marker of bone resorption and thus can also be useful in monitoring patients with metabolic bone disease. It is subject to a marked diurnal variation, so levels should be checked fasting, in the morning. Levels will also rise after a fracture and will be higher in patients with renal failure and in children and adolescents who are growing.

CHOLINESTERASE

Patients with certain mutations in the genes encoding this enzyme will experience a markedly exaggerated effect if they are administered suxamethonium, a muscle-relaxant sometimes given by anaesthetists, such that they remain paralysed for considerably longer than usual. Various forms of the enzyme can be present. Laboratory reports should aid interpretation of these results.

CREATINE KINASE (CK)

Elevations in CK are usually found in association with skeletal muscle damage. CK levels also rise after myocardial infarction, but the use of troponin testing has replaced the need to test CK in this setting. It is possible to test CK to help determine its source. The presence of the MB type suggests a cardiac origin; MM type predominates in skeletal muscle pathology. Very large increases in CK concentration are found in the clinical syndrome of rhabdomyolysis.

Occasionally, patients with rhabdomyolysis have an underlying genetic disorder predisposing to the presentation. Finding such patients can be problematic, but the following mnemonic (RHABDO)[1] is very helpful in deciding who to refer for specialist investigation:

Recurrent episodes of exertional rhabdomyolysis

HyperCK-aemia persisting 8 weeks after the event

---

[1]Scalco RS, Snoeck M, Quinlivan R, et al. Exertional rhabdomyolysis: physiological response or manifestation of an underlying myopathy? *BMJ Open Sport Exerc Med* 2016;2:e000151. doi:10.1136/bmjsem-2016-000151.

Accustomed physical exercise triggering rhabdomyolysis

Blood CK >50× the upper limit of normal

Drugs/medication/supplements and other exogenous and endogenous factors cannot sufficiently explain the rhabdomyolysis severity

Other family members affected/other exertional symptoms (cramps, myalgia)

C-REACTIVE PROTEIN (CRP)

CRP rises with most causes of inflammation (not simply infections). A patient who has a surgical procedure performed will have an elevation in CRP as a response to the surgical insult itself, and a high level of CRP in such settings does not necessary mean than an infective process is underway. The commonest use for CRP monitoring is in tracking response to anti-microbial treatment in a patient with a bacterial infection. In such circumstances, trends are generally more informative than isolated values. Bear in mind that the CRP may rise in some viral infections and in some autoimmune processes, e.g., patients with systemic lupus erythematosus. In the latter, a discrepancy between a high erythrocyte sedimentation rate (ESR) (see Chapter 15) and a relatively normal CRP may point to that diagnosis.

CRYOGLOBULINS

Cryoglobulins are proteins that precipitate out of solution when cooled and usually re-dissolve when a sample is re-warmed. Their classification is complex, and they are associated with a variety of underlying conditions, e.g., lymphoma, viral hepatitis and autoimmune diseases.

LACTATE DEHYDROGENASE (LDH)

LDH is a key enzyme involved in carbohydrate metabolism and is found in high concentrations inside many types of cell, such that damage to many types of cells will result in elevated LDH concentrations. For example, LDH was used in the past to assist in the diagnosis of myocardial infarction but is no longer used in this way because of the availability of troponin testing. It is possible to sub-classify the LDH type that is raised in a patient to try to ascertain the source, but this is rarely done. In practice, LDH can be used in combination with a series of other tests to support the diagnosis of haemolysis (see Chapter 5), and is also used for prognostication in patients with lymphoma.

MAST CELL TRYPTASE

This is most often checked when there is suspicion that a patient has had an allergic or anaphylactic event. Serial measurements following such an event will show an initial rise and then steady fall in tryptase over 24 hours following such an event.

THIOPURINE S-METHYLTRANSFERASE (TPMT)

This is most commonly tested in patients who are being considered for treatment with azathioprine (e.g., for inflammatory bowel disease) or 6-mercaptopurine (e.g. for cancer). TPMT is involved in the metabolism of these drugs. If a patient has very low (or no) activity of this enzyme, they are likely to develop bone marrow suppression when treated with these drugs.

MACRO-ENZYMES

The term 'macro-enzyme' describes an enzyme complexed with immunoglobulin. Such enzymes are found in a small number of patients and are thought to be of little clinical consequence. Their presence does, however, result in the finding of spuriously high results when the enzymes in question are tested. The most commonly occurring macro-enzymes affect prolactin (see Chapter 7), CK, LDH, AST and amylase.

Disorders of glucose

GLUCOSE

Remember that cells present in a blood sample like to eat! If a sample is delayed in getting to the laboratory, some of the glucose in the sample will be used up, and the measured result will be lower than the true result. It is now recommended that special blood tubes (containing a chemical to stop glycolysis) are used for such samples to minimise the effects of this. Glucose can be measured in whole blood on POCT analysers. For the purposes of diagnosing diabetes, and where very high or low concentrations of glucose are present, the testing of plasma glucose in a main laboratory is recommended.

Hyperglycaemia

Glucose levels are affected by eating; therefore it is important to know about the timing of the last meal when interpreting. Beware of the patient who has consumed a sugary drink in the interim! The diagnosis of diabetes mellitus and intermediate states of hyperglycaemia (i.e. not normal, but not diabetes) can be made by assessing blood glucose levels randomly, after fasting, or after an oral glucose tolerance test (OGTT). In an OGTT, a person is given a fixed amount of glucose to consume after a period of fasting, and glucose levels are checked after 2 hours. The World Health Organisation have set the cut-offs shown in Table 9.1.

Diabetes can also be diagnosed if a random glucose concentration is ≥11.1 mmol/L in someone with symptoms of the condition. If a patient has no symptoms but a glucose concentration in this range is identified, a repeat test on another occasion is necessary to make the diagnosis.

Special consideration is required for pregnant women, in whom a lower threshold is required for diagnosing gestational diabetes:

- either a fasting glucose ≥5.6 mmol/l, or
- glucose 2 hours after OGTT ≥7.8 mmol/L.

Hypoglycaemia

Low blood glucose is most commonly found as a complication of the treatment of diabetes, but there are a number of rarer causes which are important to consider (see Table 9.2).

Differentiating exogenous from endogenous insulin is important in patients who have been found to have hypoglycaemia with unsuppressed insulin levels (insulin should not be detectable when hypoglycaemia is present). A useful investigation for this purpose is measuring C-peptide. C-peptide circulates when insulin has been made by the body but not when it has been injected.

The differential diagnosis of hypoglycaemia in infants and children is much broader, as a number of metabolic diseases can present in this way.

	Fasting glucose (mmol/L)	Glucose 2 hours after OGTT (mmol/L)
Diabetes	≥7.0	≥11.1
Impaired glucose tolerance	<7.0	≥7.8 and <11.1
Impaired fasting glucose	6.1–6.9	<7.8

Table 9.1 *Defining dysglycaemic states*

Cause	Notes
Drugs	Example, insulin, sulphonylureas, alcohol
Liver disease	The liver is an important store of glycogen
Hypoadrenalism	
Kidney disease	The kidneys are involved in gluconeogenesis and
Growth hormone deficiency	insulin degradation
Insulinoma	

Table 9.2 *Common causes of hypoglycaemia*

It is usual practice to request a set of screening tests when a child has an episode of hypoglycaemia. Typical tests requested include the following:

glucose
ketones
lactate
insulin
cortisol
growth hormone
amino acids
acylcarnitine profile
urinary organic acids

These tests will diagnose many of the conditions listed above, but will also help pick up fatty acid oxidation defects, organic acidurias, and other rare conditions.

HBA1C

HbA1c is the common abbreviation for glycated haemoglobin which can be considered as a sugary variation of haemoglobin. Because red blood cells containing haemoglobin circulate for approximately 3 months, HbA1c provides a useful metric of the average glucose concentration during that timeframe. HbA1c is most often used for monitoring control in a patient with diabetes, but it can also be used for diagnosing type 2 diabetes in some adults. An HbA1c ≥48 mmol/mol confirmed on two samples should be present to make the diagnosis of type 2 diabetes. This approach to diagnosis is not appropriate in pregnant women, in those with pancreatic disease, in those who are acutely unwell or taking some medications and in people in whom the HbA1c measurement may be unreliable. The measurement of fructosamine can be helpful in patients whose red blood cells have a shortened lifespan.

KETONES

Ketones are produced during fat metabolism. They are measured in several main circumstances:

- Diagnosis and monitoring of diabetic ketoacidosis.
- Investigation of high anion gap metabolic acidosis.
- Investigation of hypoglycaemia (especially in children). The normal response to hypoglycaemia is the production of ketones. Insufficient ketone production in this context may suggest a fatty acid oxidation defect.

CHAPTER 10

Lipids and other tests relevant to cardiovascular disease

LIPIDS

Everyone's level of circulating triglyceride rises after a meal containing fat as the body transports fat from the intestine. Samples for triglyceride analysis should therefore be performed fasting.

A common difficulty when trying to interpret lipid profiles is that the information provided is different to what is covered when reading about lipid physiology. We will spend a little time considering what is measured now.

The following is generally reported on a lipid profile:
- total cholesterol
- triglyceride
- high-density lipoprotein (HDL) cholesterol
- low-density lipoprotein (LDL) cholesterol
- cholesterol: HDL ratio
- non-HDL cholesterol

While the following lipid particles (lipoproteins) are often referred to when discussing lipid metabolism:
- HDL particles (of various types)
- intermediate-density lipoprotein particles

- LDL particles
- very-low-density lipoprotein (VLDL) particles
- chylomicron remnants
- chylomicrons

Lipoproteins differ in terms of their lipid composition and surface proteins (known as apolipoproteins). Chylomicrons, chylomicron remnants and VLDL have relatively more triglyceride then cholesterol, whereas IDL, LDL and HDL have proportionally more cholesterol. Whilst it is possible to measure the quantities of each lipoprotein in the laboratory using techniques such as ultracentrifugation and electrophoresis, these techniques are highly labour-intensive and are not suitable for most clinical laboratories.

Total cholesterol

When interpreting this result, it is helpful to imagine that the lipoproteins have been put in a blender by the laboratory (they have not, but it is a useful analogy!). The total amount of cholesterol present (both free and esterified) is then measured, but there is no easy way of telling from which lipoproteins the cholesterol has originated. Total cholesterol measurements are therefore of limited utility, although widely quoted in the lay literature and familiar to many patients.

Triglyceride

As for total cholesterol, imagine that the serum or plasma has been blended. The total amount of triglyceride present is then measured, but there is no easy way of telling from which lipoproteins it has originated. Very high concentrations of triglycerides in samples are usually due to either the presence of high quantities of VLDL lipoproteins and/or chylomicrons. A useful qualitative test can be done to differentiate between these. The specimen tube should be stored upright in a laboratory refrigerator for up to 24 hours (overnight usually suffices). If chylomicrons are present, a creamy layer will float to the top (much like the head on a pint of Guinness!). If VLDL is present in high quantities, the serum/plasma will be turbid. See Fig. 10.1 for an example.

HDL-cholesterol

Imagine that the laboratory puts the sample through a special filter which only lets HDL through. The total cholesterol content of the HDL passing through the filter is then measured.

LDL-cholesterol

It has traditionally been challenging to measure LDL-cholesterol directly in the laboratory, although new methods are being developed for this

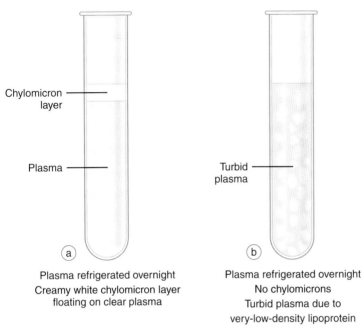

Chylomicron
layer

Plasma

Turbid
plasma

(a)

(b)

Plasma refrigerated overnight
Creamy white chylomicron layer
floating on clear plasma

Plasma refrigerated overnight
No chylomicrons
Turbid plasma due to
very-low-density lipoprotein

Fig.10.1   *Identifying chylomicrons in lipaemic samples*

purpose. In most laboratories, an estimate of LDL is provided using an equation known as the Friedewald equation. This equation first estimates the VLDL concentration in the sample by dividing the triglyceride result by a constant. It then estimates LDL concentration by subtracting measured HDL and estimated VLDL from the total cholesterol result. The equation is not accurate when triglycerides are high (>4.7 mmol/L), and does not perform well in some patients with genetic lipid disorders. You will commonly see 'Not reportable' listed for LDL in patients in whom the triglyceride concentration is high.

Cholesterol:HDL ratio

This is simply the total cholesterol concentration divided by the HDL concentration.

Non-HDL cholesterol

This is simply total cholesterol minus HDL cholesterol.

Interpreting the results

Although reference ranges are provided for lipid results and are useful for interpreting triglyceride levels, results for cholesterol are most often interpreted in conjunction with clinical risk prediction algorithms and in conjunction with guidelines from expert groups. In the UK for example, a patient who has never suffered a cardiovascular event, will often have their cardiovascular risk estimated using a calculator like QRISK3 (https://qrisk.org/three/) which incorporates the cholesterol: HDL ratio. A decision on whether or not to treat their cholesterol will be made by interpreting this risk in light of guidelines from the National Institute for Health and Care Excellence (NICE). NICE also set cost-effective treatment targets which are useful for those on treatment, and presently quote targets for non-HDL cholesterol reduction.

Generic risk predicting tools are very helpful for the bulk of the population, but should not be used in certain patients such as those with genetic disorders of lipid metabolism.

Other lipid tests

Apolipoprotein A-1 (Apo-A1)

This is the principal protein found on the surface of HDL lipoproteins. Measuring this provides another estimate of the amount of circulating HDL. This test is currently not performed routinely.

Apolipoprotein B (Apo B)

There are two main forms of Apo B – B48 and B100. Apo B48 is found on the surface of chylomicrons, whereas Apo B100 is associated with VLDL. Measuring either of these proteins can provide an estimate of the respective lipoproteins in the sample. This test is currently not performed routinely.

Lipoprotein(a) (Lp(a))

Lp(a), affectionately referred to as 'lipoprotein little a', is another circulating lipoprotein which is gaining traction as being of high importance in the pathogenesis of atherosclerosis in some individuals. The higher the measured concentration, the higher the risk for that individual.

OTHER TESTS RELEVANT TO CARDIOVASCULAR DISEASE

Cardiac troponin

In the past, various proteins were tested in an attempt to detect myocardial damage, e.g., aspartate aminotransferase, lactate dehydrogenase, and creatine kinase. Due to much improved sensitivity and specificity, however, these tests have all been replaced by measurement of troponin I or T. The definition of myocardial injury and myocardial infarction has become rather complex, but central to the 'universal definition' is the finding of elevated cardiac troponin values with at least one value above the 99th percentile upper reference limit.[1] Acute myocardial injury is deemed to be present when troponin rises and/or falls. Signs and/or symptoms of clinical myocardial ischaemia must be present to make a diagnosis of acute myocardial infarction.

Cardiac troponin may be elevated for reasons other than myocardial injury, a small number of which are shown in Table 10.1.

B-type natriuretic peptide (BNP)

There are several variations of this test in common use, but all are used for the same purpose – screening for or monitoring of heart failure. BNP is released from the ventricles of the heart when they are stretched, and in a patient suspected of having heart failure, the test is excellent at ruling this condition out if a normal result is returned. Conditions other than heart failure can, however, increase BNP levels, as shown in Table 10.2.

Myocardial injury/infarction
Pulmonary embolism
Sepsis
Aortic dissection
Endocarditis

Table 10.1 *Common causes of elevated cardiac troponin*

Heart failure
Any condition causing hypoxia, e.g., pulmonary embolism
Atrial fibrillation
Kidney disease
Liver disease

Table 10.2 *Common causes of elevated BNP*

[1]Thygesen, K et al., (2019). Fourth universal definition of myocardial infarction. *European Heart Journal* 40, 237–269.

Tumour markers

THE USE OF TUMOUR MARKERS

Blood tumour markers are tests which, when present in higher than normal concentration, can be associated with cancer. They can be used to:

- diagnose cancer
- prognosticate
- track progress and response to treatment

Used properly, tumour markers are very useful tests, but appropriate requesting is necessary, as is an appreciation of the inherent problems with these tests. Table 11.1 details the tumour markers in widespread use. Consider the following when interpreting these results.

Is the result really normal or abnormal?

You may wish to refer to the description of reference ranges in Chapter 2 at this stage. Consider testing for the presence of a particular tumour marker in a large number of people known to have a particular type of cancer and a large number of people who do not have it. If we plot how often a particular result crops up in the two groups of people, something like what is shown in Fig.11.1 might be found.

If we then go on to test three patients, we can plot their results on this chart in an attempt to make a diagnosis. Patient 1's result suggests that he/she is unlikely to have cancer. Patient 2's result suggests that they are highly likely to have cancer. Patient 3's results are harder to interpret, being somewhere in the overlap zone between the two disease states.

Tumour Marker	Associated Tumour
Alpha fetoprotein (AFP)	Germ cell Hepatocellular carcinoma
Calcitonin	Medullary cell thyroid
Carbohydrate antigen 19-9 (CA19-9)	Pancreas
Carbohydrate antigen 125 (CA-125)	Ovary
Carbohydrate antigen 15-3 (CA15-3)	Breast
Carcinoembryonic antigen (CEA)	Colorectal
Chromogranin A (CgA)*	Any neuroendocrine tumour
Human chorionic gonadotrophin (HCG)	Choriocarcinoma Germ cell
Free metanephrines	Phaeochromocytoma and paraganglioma
5-hydroxyindoleacetic acid (HIAA)	Carcinoid syndrome
Paraprotein	Multiple myeloma
Prostate specific antigen (PSA)	Prostate
Thyroglobulin	Follicular thyroid Papillary thyroid

*Neuroendocrine tumours are rare and secrete hormones depending on their particular type. All such tumours (including carcinoid tumours also shown separately in the table) tend to release chromogranin A, which is non-specific. More specific testing for neuroendocrine tumours is generally selected based on the clinical presentation.

Table 11.1 *Commonly requested tumour markers*

Sometimes, cut-off values or decision levels are made to aid in the interpretation of a tumour result. For our example, consider the effects of introducing a cut-off at three different levels, illustrated in Fig.11.2.

If cut-off 1 is chosen to signify a result worthy of further investigation for cancer, all cancers will be picked up, but a large number of people who do not have cancer will be sent for further testing. At this cut-off level, the test could be said to be sensitive but not specific. If cut-off 3 is chosen, all patients with a positive test will have cancer, but a large proportion of patients with cancer will be missed. The test would then be specific but not sensitive. Cut-off 2 lies somewhere in between. A small number of

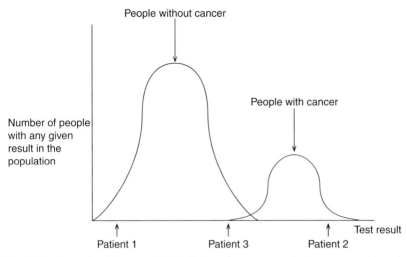

Fig.11.1 *Example of the potential distribution of a tumour marker in a group with and without cancer*

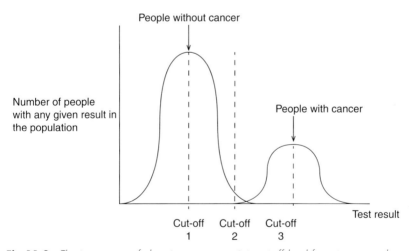

Fig.11.2 *The importance of choosing an appropriate cut-off level for a tumour marker*

people without cancer would require further testing if they had a result at this level, and a small number of people with cancer will be missed. Cut-offs for cancer are usually chosen in such a way that they aim to not miss a person with cancer and that they minimise misclassification of a person who does not have cancer. No tumour marker is perfect, and there will always be false positives (people who have 'high' values of a tumour marker but do not have cancer) and false negatives (people who have 'low' values but do have cancer).

Is something other than cancer affecting a result?

For many tumour markers, there is a long list of conditions other than cancer that can cause an elevated result. Take prostatic specific antigen (PSA) for example. Infection in the prostate gland or elsewhere in the urinary tract, or a recent digital rectal examination can all elevate PSA for a short time and may cause confusion.

Trends are often more informative than one-off values

As with many blood tests (see Chapter 2), the pattern of change for a tumour marker with time is often much more informative than a one-off result with no context. Thus, a patient who is being followed up for recurrence of a cancer, who has a steadily rising tumour marker, is clearly in a different position to a patient receiving cancer treatment whose tumour marker is falling.

Nutrition

IRON

An iron profile typically comprises the following tests:
1. Iron—a measure of the circulating iron. This is generally not a very useful test, as levels fluctuate during the course of a day and rise after acute iron ingestion.
2. Total iron-binding capacity (TIBC)—an indirect measure of the transferrin (iron-carrying protein) concentration.
3. Transferrin saturation—calculated (not measured) as the ratio of iron to TIBC.
4. Ferritin—a measure of iron stores. Ferritin behaves as an acute-phase reactant (like C-reactive protein), and levels will rise in the setting of acute inflammation, making it more difficult to interpret in such settings.

Clinical reasons for requesting an iron profile:
1. Iron deficiency—expect to find:
   a. high TIBC (the body trying to grab hold of any available iron)
   b. low transferrin saturation
   c. low ferritin (unless there is acute inflammation)
2. Iron overload in haemochromatosis—expect to find:
   a. high transferrin saturation
   b. high ferritin

3. To diagnose or monitor a disease associated with very high ferritin concentrations, e.g., adult-onset Still's disease, severe COVID-19, or haemophagocytic lymphohistiocytosis.
4. Acute iron poisoning:
   a. serum iron levels will guide treatment decisions

A common cause for confusion is the appearance of the iron profile in patients who have anaemia of chronic disease. Typically, TIBC will be low and ferritin normal or raised.

More specialised tests (e.g., soluble transferrin factors) can be performed in more difficult cases.

FOLATE

Folate results are straightforward to interpret – low, normal or high.

VITAMIN B12

The laboratory assessment of true vitamin B12 status is complex, as what is measured as 'vitamin B12' is not the active substance. Thus, patients can be truly vitamin B12 deficient with a normal blood level; therefore a high degree of suspicion is required, particularly in patients whose blood level is towards the lower end of the reference range. Other tests may be helpful in ascertaining true vitamin B12 status:
- Holotranscobalamin—this is, effectively, 'active' B12, and a low level suggests deficiency.
- Methylmalonic acid (MMA)—levels rise in B12 deficiency.
- Total homocysteine—levels rise in B12 deficiency, but a rise is also seen in folate deficiency, cigarette smoking, and other situations. Very high levels suggest the possibility of the inherited metabolic disease, homocystinuria.

MICRONUTRIENT SCREEN

There is a large number of micronutrients, and many can be tested in blood. Often testing of 'micronutrient panel' will be provided by a laboratory. Such a screen might include measurement of the following, in addition to those tests listed earlier:
- Vitamin A
- Vitamin C
- Vitamin E
- Selenium: This is most often requested in the monitoring of patients on special diets or at particular risk of deficiency.

- Copper: This is most often requested in the assessment of possible Wilson's disease (where it is not as helpful as other metrics of copper metabolism, see Chapter 5) and in monitoring patients on special diets or at particular risk of deficiency. When interpreting results, bear in mind that high oestrogen states (e.g., pregnancy, use of an oral contraceptive pill) increase copper levels.
- Zinc: This is most often requested in the monitoring of patients on special diets or at particular risk of deficiency. Zinc levels fall in situations of acute inflammation.

MAGNESIUM

Contamination of a sample with EDTA can cause a falsely low level of magnesium (see Chapter 2). Like potassium, the body's magnesium handling can be considered as in Fig. 12.1.

High levels of magnesium are usually due to too much magnesium being administered to a patient. Common causes of hypomagnesaemia are shown in Table 12.1.

VITAMIN D

Testing of vitamin D has become a very frequent test, but in many cases it is unnecessary. Interpretation of results is easy, with results generally being classified as 'deficient', 'insufficient' or 'sufficient.' Severe vitamin D deficiency is associated with rickets (in children) and osteomalacia (in adults) – see Chapter 4. Note that it is usually 25(OH)-vitamin D that is measured, rather than calcitriol.

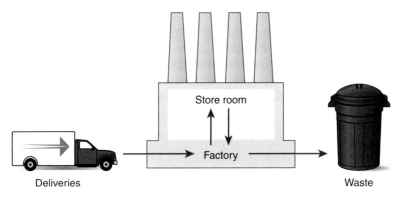

Fig.12.1 *A simple model of a factory which can assist in understanding some electrolyte abnormalities*

Too little in	Chronic malnutrition Use of proton pump inhibitors (block absorption)
Shift from blood into cells	Re-feeding syndrome Treatment of diabetic ketoacidosis
Too much out	Diarrhoea Inflammatory bowel disease Diuretics Alcoholism (increases renal losses)

Table 12.1 *Common causes of hypomagnesaemia*

URATE

Urate is produced as a result of purine metabolism, and a high circulating level is associated with gout. Urate levels may be high on account of rapid cell turnover (e.g., some cancers, cell lysis syndrome), increased production (e.g., due to a rare metabolic disorder) or reduced excretion (e.g., chronic kidney disease, thiazide diuretics). Interpretation of urate levels during an episode of acute gout may be complicated by the fact that urate levels can fall during an attack.

Therapeutic drug monitoring and toxicology

THERAPEUTIC DRUG MONITORING (TDM)

TDM (measuring levels of therapeutic drugs in bodily fluids, most commonly blood) is undertaken for several reasons:

- Assessing concordance. If a patient says that they are taking a drug, but none can be detected in the system, then they should be challenged again.
- Looking for toxicity. A drug may need to be stopped or have its dose reduced if levels are too high.
- Ensuring that a therapeutic level has been reached. Some drugs are not effective unless a certain blood level is reached.

Perfectly healthy people do not need to take medication; therefore the concept of a 'reference range' does not apply to TDM, as the drug will not be detected unless someone has been taking it. Instead, the concept of a 'therapeutic range' is important. For example, if a drug is ineffective below a concentration of 'a' mg/L and is toxic above a concentration of 'b' mg/L, then the therapeutic range is 'a to b'. A drug with a small difference between being ineffective and being toxic is said to have a narrow therapeutic range. This is illustrated in Fig. 13.1.

Knowledge of how blood levels of drugs varies with time is the basis of the science of pharmacokinetics, and a detailed knowledge of this is not required for most people who are interpreting TDM results. A few core principles are, however, useful to remember:

- If a patient is established on an intravenous infusion of a drug which is being given at a continuous rate perfectly matched to the drug's clearance from the body, a straight horizontal line will be obtained if blood

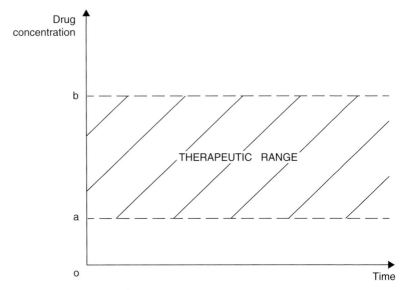

Fig. 13.1 *The concept of 'therapeutic range'*

levels are plotted with time. This is very rarely the case for most drugs in clinical practice.

– For patients who are administered drugs intermittently, the blood level of the drug will vary with time. An example is shown in Fig. 13.2.

Looking at Fig. 13.2, you will note that it takes several doses of a drug before a consistent pattern of blood levels is obtained. This is dependent on a property of a drug known as its half-life. You will also note that peak drug levels are present shortly after dosing (or immediately if the drug is given intravenously), and that trough levels are present just prior to the next dose. Knowing the timing of a TDM sample and the timing of the administration of the drug in question is therefore critical when interpreting TDM results. For some drugs, trough levels are most important; for others, levels should be checked at a set time after drug administration. Details on the best timing for samples is best obtained from your local laboratory. Drugs commonly measured in TDM are listed in Table 13.1.

TOXICOLOGY

Drugs of abuse

Drugs of abuse screening is often performed in patients who are drowsy under suspicious circumstances, or at the request of a team monitoring a patient with a previous addiction. Panels of tests are usually performed. The usual approach

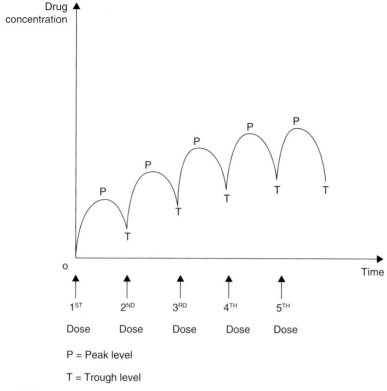

Fig. 13.2 *Blood drug concentration after serial administration*

is to screen for a particular class of drug. More detailed testing can then be performed if required. For example, a urinary screen may indicate the presence of 'opiates', but a specific test will be required to identify which opiates are present.

Specific poisons

It is possible to test the blood level of a large number of potential poisons, and management guidelines are often dependent upon the levels measured. Interpretation of such results is usually fairly straightforward – deciding to send the test is most challenging.

Paracetamol

It is vital that paracetamol toxicity is detected early so that the institution of appropriate antidote therapy can be administered to the patient. In acute paracetamol poisoning, it is imperative that paracetamol levels are checked

Drug class	Examples	Notes
Anti-convulsants	Phenytoin	Due to unusual metabolism, small changes in dosing can have large effects on levels
	Carbamazepine Valproate Lamotrigine Levetiracetam Phenobarbitone	Toxicity is seen with some of these drugs, but levels are often checked to ensure that a patient with seemingly resistant epilepsy is concordant with their treatment
	Thiopentone	Sometimes used in intensive care units. Levels often checked after administration stopped to determine when low levels of the drug are present so that testing for brainstem death can be performed
Immunosuppressants	Ciclosporin Everolimus Methotrexate Mycophenolate Sirolimus Tacrolimus	
Anti-microbials	Gentamicin Amikacin Vancomycin Tobramycin Teicoplanin	
Anti-arrhythmics	Digoxin	
Other	Lithium	Falsely high levels will be obtained if samples are collected in a lithium-heparin tube
	Prednisolone Theophylline	

Table 13.1 *Drugs commonly measured in the laboratory*

at least 4 hours after ingestion of the drug. Once a level is measured, proceed to plot the paracetamol level on a nomogram such as the one shown in Fig.13.3. If the measured level is above the decision line, the patient should receive antidote treatment.

Left untreated, paracetamol poisoning can cause liver failure, kidney failure and lactic acidosis.

Salicylate

Poisoning with aspirin can be confirmed on a blood test for salicylate, but the manifestations of aspirin poisoning may be suspected for other reasons.

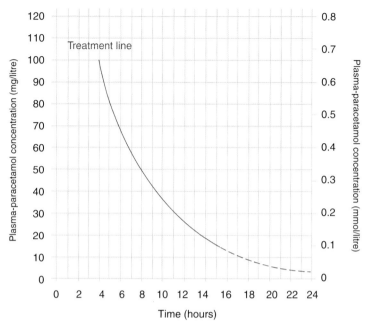

Fig. 13.3 *Paracetamol toxicity nomogram*

Salicylate poisoning triggers a respiratory alkalosis (as the respiratory centre is stimulated) and a co-existent metabolic acidosis.

Toxic alcohols

So-called 'toxic alcohols' include methanol and ethylene glycol. Sometimes patients volunteer that they have ingested such substances, but quite often they are reluctant to provide this information. In such instances, a high index of suspicion is required. Clues to this diagnosis include the following:

1. Osmolar gap: Calculate the estimated serum osmolality using the formula provided in Chapter 3. Next, obtain a laboratory measure of osmolality and calculate the 'osmolar gap' (also described in Chapter 3). A significantly raised gap is in keeping with the ingestion of a toxic alcohol. Note that this gap would be expected to decrease with time.
2. High anion gap metabolic acidosis (see Chapter 6).
3. High lactate gap: This is the difference between the blood lactate level measured in a POCT analyser and that measured in a main laboratory. Results should be fairly similar, but in ethylene glycol poisoning, an error can occur in the POCT analyser, resulting in the lactate gap.

Once suspected, blood can be checked for the presence of a toxic alcohol, but this process is labour-intensive.

Digoxin

Pay attention to potassium results when digoxin toxicity is identified, as potassium abnormalities make complications with digoxin more likely.

Carbon monoxide

See Chapter 6.

Metabolic testing

With the exception of ammonia, lactate and a screening test for porphyria, ordering and interpreting metabolic tests is usually restricted to chemical pathologists and paediatricians who treat children with inherited metabolic diseases. As such, only superficial coverage of some of these topics is presented here.

AMMONIA

Ammonia is a nitrogen-containing compound that is generated from various sources in the body:
- breakdown of protein and amino acids
- the action of gut bacteria
- muscle metabolism
- kidney metabolism

Moderate hyperammonaemia can be spurious, but aside from this, in adults, the vast majority of cases of hyperammonaemia arise in the context of liver failure. The liver has a key role in clearing ammonia from the blood, and in many liver diseases, vascular shunting occurs such that ammonia being generated in the gut is directly transferred into the systemic circulation. There is also a large number of uncommon causes of hyperammonaemia, therefore the scheme in Fig. 14.1 should be helpful in working up a patient with this problem. The main alternative conditions to think about in adults are: urinary tract infection with an organism that expresses urease

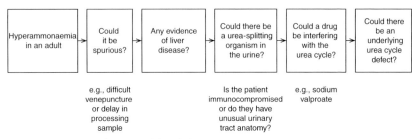

Fig. 14.1 *Approach to an adult with hyperammonaemia*

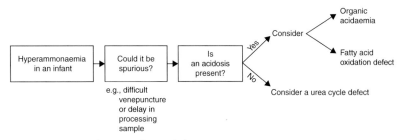

Fig. 14.2 *Approach to an infant with hyperammonaemia*

(generates ammonia from urea), a drug that is interfering with the normal handling of ammonia, or an undiagnosed fault in the metabolic pathway that handles ammonia, the urea cycle.

Urea cycle disorders are rare, and there are several types. Differentiating between them is a job for a specialist in this field and requires testing of intermediate compounds in the cycle.

In infants, hyperammonaemia is much more likely to be due to a serious underlying metabolic defect than in adulthood. A suggested approach to the problem is shown in Fig. 14.2. Investigating these rare disorders should be carried out by a specialist.

LACTATE

Lactate is requested very frequently in acutely unwell patients, and should additionally be checked in all patients with a high anion gap metabolic acidosis (see Chapter 6). It is the end-product of anaerobic metabolism, and in the vast majority of cases, the cause is obvious: either the patient is hypoxic, and there is insufficient oxygen being delivered to cells for them to undertake aerobic respiration, or the patient has circulatory collapse and the oxygen is not delivered properly to the cells, with the same metabolic outcome. In other cases, there may be a problem with delivering oxygen to a specific organ, e.g., the cells in an acutely ischaemic limb or segment of bowel will produce lactate. Lactate is often raised after an epileptic

Mechanism	Example
Hypoxia	Respiratory failure Carbon monoxide poisoning Anaemia
Hypoperfusion	Septic shock Cardiogenic shock Embolism
Extreme muscular activity	Status epilepticus
Severe organ dysfunction	Liver failure Kidney failure
Drug-induced	Metformin Paracetamol poisoning Toxic alcohol ingestion
Inherited metabolic disease	Fatty acid oxidation defect Organic aciduria Disorder affecting glycolysis pathway

Table 14.1 *Causes of elevated lactate*

seizure due to the vigorous muscle activity. Causes of elevated lactate are listed in Table 14.1.

Further testing to identify the cause of a high lactate concentration may be necessary, if not clear from the clinical presentation.

D-lactate

The (common) lactate referred to above is L-lactate. D-lactate must be tested for specifically. D-lactate is produced in some patients with short bowel syndrome as carbohydrates are not fully absorbed in the short bowel and can reach the colon where bacteria act on them thus forming D-lactate. D-lactate is an uncommon cause of a high anion gap metabolic acidosis.

PORPHYRINS AND RELATED COMPOUNDS

The porphyrias are a group of disorders that result because of a problem in the metabolic pathway that generates haem, the iron-containing compound found in haemoglobin. Differentiating between the various disorders relies on an assessment of clinical features and on interpretation of blood, urine and faeces laboratory test results, and is the job of a specialist in this field. The key test for diagnosing an acute hepatic attack of porphyria is not a blood test – it is urinary porphobilinogen (PBG). If PBG is elevated, further laboratory testing is necessary to diagnose the subtype of porphyria present. All samples being sent to a laboratory in relation to porphyria testing must be protected from light.

ACYLCARNITINES

Acylcarnitines are intermediate compounds formed in mitochondria during energy generation from fatty acids. There are a large number of rare metabolic diseases, collectively known as fatty acid oxidation defects. Each is associated with a particular pattern of abnormalities in acylcarnitines. The commonest of such conditions is medium chain acyl-coenzyme A dehydrogenase deficiency (MCADD).

AMINO ACIDS

It is possible to test for all standard amino acids, and such testing is performed routinely in patients with certain inherited metabolic diseases that affect certain amino acid levels and that require specialist dietetic treatment. Each relevant disease produces characteristic patterns of abnormalities on amino acid testing. The commonest disorder with characteristic results is phenylketonuria (PKU). Patients with this condition have very high circulating levels of phenylalanine. Intake of dietary protein and amino acids will have a bearing on measured amino acid levels.

NEWBORN BLOOD SCREENING

All newborn babies are offered (subject to parental consent) a screening blood test, usually around day 5 of life. Capillary blood is sampled from the infant's heel. Testing is performed in specialist laboratories and according to agreed protocols that vary by country. The hard work for these tests is performed in the laboratory. The requestor simply must interpret a fairly straightforward set of results that generally state that condition X is either suspected or not suspected. If a disease is suspected, further confirmatory tests are undertaken.

OTHER METABOLIC TESTS

Because of the vast number of metabolic pathways that exist in the body, there are a huge number of rare metabolic diseases. Advances in laboratory testing in recent decades has opened up the ability to diagnose many of these conditions. Knowledge of such tests is not necessary for most healthcare professionals.

The full blood picture (FBP)

The full blood picture (also called 'full blood count' or 'complete blood count') provides lots of information about the circulating cell types, as detailed in Table 15.1. Most information can be gleaned from the study of the five parameters highlighted in bold.

HAEMOGLOBIN

Imagine that the red blood cells are put through a 'blender' in the laboratory, so that all the haemoglobin escapes. The concentration is then measured. The chief purpose for assessing haemoglobin concentration is to allow the detection of anaemia. Anaemia is defined as a low haemoglobin concentration below set cut-offs as determined by the World Health Organisation and shown in Table 15.2.

MEAN CELL VOLUME

Mean cell volume (MCV) is an average of the volume of red blood cells. People who consume alcohol in excess often have a high MCV (see Chapter 5), but the most useful application of MCV is in the assessment of a patient with anaemia, as the main causes for anaemia can be sub-divided depending on the MCV result, as shown in Table 15.3.

Test	Abbreviation	What it means
Haemoglobin concentration	Hb	The amount of haemoglobin in a specified volume once cell membranes have been disrupted
Red blood cell count	RBC	Number of red blood cells in a specified volume
Haematocrit	HCT	The proportion of the blood volume taken up by red blood cells
Mean cell volume	MCV	The average volume of red blood cells in the sample
Mean cell haemoglobin	MCH	The average amount of haemoglobin in each red blood cell
Mean cell haemoglobin concentration	MCHC	The average concentration of haemoglobin in each red blood cell
Red cell distribution width	RDW	A measure of the variation in size of red blood cells. High RDW may indicate dual pathology
Platelet count	Plt	Number of platelets in a specified volume
Leucocyte count	WBC	Number of white blood cells (leucocytes) in a specified volume
Neutrophils	Neutr	Number of neutrophils in a specified volume
Lymphocytes	Lymph	Number of lymphocytes in a specified volume
Monocytes	Mono	Number of monocytes in a specified volume
Eosinophils	Eos	Number of eosinophils in a specified volume
Basophils	Baso	Number of basophils in a specified volume
Reticulocytes	Retic	Number of reticulocytes (immature red cells) in a specified volume

Table 15.1 *Constituent parts of the full blood picture*

Group	Threshold for diagnosing anaemia (g/L)
Men	130
Non-pregnant women	120
Pregnant women	110

Table 15.2 *Diagnosis of anaemia*

MCV result	Anaemia classification	Common causes
Low	Microcytic	Iron deficiency Thalassaemia Chronic disease
Normal	Normocytic	Chronic disease Acute bleeding Haemolytic anaemia
High	Macrocytic	Folate deficiency Vitamin B12 deficiency

Table 15.3 *Mean cell volume interpretation*

You will hear the term 'megaloblastic anaemia' being used frequently. This term can be used in patients with macrocytic anaemia when megaloblasts (immature red cells) are seen in bone marrow.

HAEMATOCRIT

Haematocrit (HCT) is the proportion of the blood volume taken up by red blood cells. When a blood sample is spun in a centrifuge, the red cells sink to the bottom (see 'plasma' part of Fig. 2.1 in Chapter 2). A blood sample with a higher red blood cell mass will have a higher haematocrit. The main purpose of checking HCT is to identify polycythaemia. Guidelines have been drawn up for the investigation of patients with persistently raised HCT (>0.52 for males, >0.48 for females). Polycythaemia can be a problem in its own right (polycythaemia vera), or secondary to an underlying condition, e.g., hypoxia or abnormal erythropoietin production.

LEUCOCYTE COUNT

Haematology laboratories use a variety of techniques to count the different types of white blood cells (leucocytes). Common white cell count abnormalities are shown in Table 15.4.

	Low	High
Neutrophils	Viral infection Drug-induced, e.g., clozapine	Bacterial infection Inflammation Tissue necrosis
Lymphocytes	Often non-specific finding Infections including HIV	Viral infection Lymphocytic leukaemia
Monocytes	–	Chronic infection
Eosinophils	–	Hypersensitivity disorders Parasitic infections
Basophils	–	Myeloproliferative disorders

Table 15.4 *Common white cell abnormalities and their causes*

In patients with infections, following the trend in leucocyte count is almost always more useful than interpreting one result in isolation (see Chapter 2 for more details).

PLATELET COUNT

Common important causes of both low (thrombocytopaenia) and high (thrombocytosis) platelet counts are shown in Table 15.5.

APPROACH TO A PATIENT WITH ANAEMIA

There are a number of ways of classifying anaemia. You might find Fig. 15.1 helpful when considering an anaemic patient.

Fig. 15.2 should help you classify the anaemia and plan a useful set of investigations to delve deeper. Remember that finding a cause for the anaemia is only part of making a complete diagnosis in many patients. Additionally, you should try to 'find a cause for the cause.' For example, a patient with microcytic anaemia might have iron deficiency anaemia caused by a tumour in their colon, a patient with vitamin B12 deficiency might have Crohn's disease, and there are many causes of haemolytic anaemia. Whole guidelines have been written to assist in the investigation and management of patients with anaemia of different causes.

In haemolytic anaemia, the bilirubin concentration will rise due to haemoglobin breakdown, increased amounts of circulating enzymes normally found in red cells, e.g., lactate dehydrogenase and aspartate aminotransferase will be detected, and low concentrations of haptoglobin (a protein that mops up haemoglobin) would be expected.

Thrombocytopaenia	Thrombocytosis
Immune thrombocytopenic purpura	Essential thrombocythaemia Active bleeding Inflammation Malignant cancer

Table 15.5 *Common causes of an abnormal platelet count*

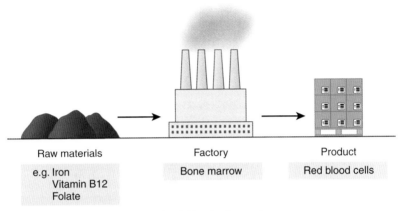

Raw materials — e.g. Iron, Vitamin B12, Folate

Factory — Bone marrow

Product — Red blood cells

Fig. 15.1 *A schematic representation of red blood cell manufacture*

APPROACH TO A PATIENT WITH AN ELEVATED HAEMATOCRIT

There are a range of causes for persistently elevated HCT, but in general terms, patients may have a primary problem where they produce excessive quantities of red blood cells (polycythaemia vera) or a secondary problem associated with increased erythropoietin (EPO) production (e.g., hypoxia, or an EPO-producing tumour). Fig. 15.3 offers an initial approach for the investigation of this problem. This is based on a published guideline,[1] and interested readers are encouraged to read the guideline in full for more information.

BLOOD FILM INTERPRETATION

When a sample of whole blood is spread out on a slide and examined under a microscope, a detailed assessment of the shape of the cells present can

---

[1]McMullin M F *et al* (2018). A guideline for the diagnosis and management of polycythaemia vera. A British Society for Haematology Guideline. *British Journal of Haematology* 184, 176–191.

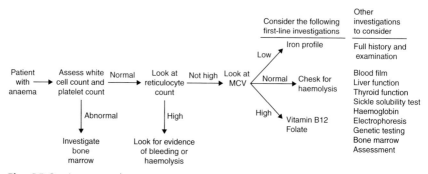

Fig. 15.2 *An approach to investigating anaemia*

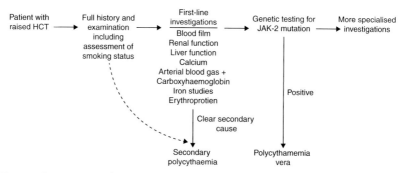

Fig. 15.3 *An approach to a patient with an elevated haematocrit*

be made. Characteristic shapes are seen in some diseases. Interpretation of blood films is normally carried out by a haematologist, such that a written report is prepared for the requestor. It is important to be able to understand the terminology that is used in these reports. Common terms are listed in Table 15.6. Interested readers may wish to look up the appearance of these abnormalities online.

ERYTHROCYTE SEDIMENTATION RATE (ESR)

ESR is a measure of the settlement of red blood cells in a thin column of blood over a set time period (without the use of a centrifuge). During periods of inflammation, the presence of increased amounts of circulating proteins in a sample means that the cells settle quicker and the ESR will be higher.

Name of abnormality	Description	Example causes
Abnormal red cells		
Shape		
Acanthocyte	Red cell with irregular spikes on its surface	Splenectomy, liver disease
Dacrocyte (tear drop cell)	Red cells that resemble tears or droplets of water	Myelofibrosis
Echinocyte (burr cell)	Red cell with regular spikes on its surface	Delayed processing, liver failure, kidney failure
Elliptocyte (pencil cell)	Long, thin red cell	Iron deficiency
Keratocyte	Horned red cell (looks like a bite has been taken out of the cell)	Microangiopathic haemolytic anaemia
Ovalocyte	Red cell with oval shape	B12 and folate deficiency
Poikilocytosis	Abnormal shapes of red cells	Iron deficiency
Schistocyte	Irregularly shaped fragment of a destroyed red cell	Microangiopathic haemolytic anaemia
Sickle cell	Red cells that resemble sickles (a tool with a curved blade)	Sickle cell disease
Spherocyte	Red cells that are spherical (recognised by lack of central pale area)	Hereditary spherocytosis
Stomatocyte	Red cell with mouth-shaped central pale area	Alcohol excess
Target cell	Red cells that resemble targets	Thalassaemia
Size		
Anisocytosis	Differing sizes of red cells	Vitamin B12 or folate deficiency
Colour		
Anisochromia	Pale red cells	Iron deficiency
Hypochromic	Differing colour of red cells due to premature release from bone marrow	Anaemia
Polychromatic	Differing density of colour of red cells	Post-transfusion
Content		
Basophilic stippling	Blue RNA granules in cytoplasm of red cells	Lead poisoning
Heinz bodies	Denatured haemoglobin seen as clumps within red cells	Thalassaemia
Howell-Jolly bodies	Dot inside red blood cell (due to a nucleus)	Splenectomy
Pappenheimer bodies	Granules of iron inside red cells	Myelodysplastic syndrome
Trophozoites	Small dots inside red blood cells (due to the presence of a parasite)	Malaria (*Plasmodium falciparum*)

Table 15.6 *Terms used in blood film reports—cont'd*

Name of abnormality	Description	Example causes
Abnormal white cells		
Overall appearance		
Blast cells	Abnormal, immature white cells	Leukaemia
Smear cells	Lymphocytes with ruptured cell membranes (rupturing happens when preparing a blood film for examination)	Chronic lymphocytic leukaemia
Content		
Auer rods	Needle-like granular material inside blast cells	Acute myeloid leukaemia
Döhle bodies	Small blue-grey bodies inside neutrophils	Severe inflammation e.g., in sepsis
Hypersegmented neutrophil	Six or more segments visible in neutrophil nucleus	Vitamin B12 or folate deficiency
Toxic granulation of neutrophil	Large granules in cytoplasm of neutrophils	Severe inflammation e.g., in sepsis
Abnormalities in several cell types		
Leucoerythroblastic blood picture	Immature red cells, white cells and platelets	Severe sepsis, bone marrow infiltration

Table 15.6 *Terms used in blood film reports*

Tests of coagulation

A standard 'coagulation screen' provides the following, shown in Table 16.1.

PROTHROMBIN TIME (PT)

Chemicals are added to a blood sample, and the time taken to clot is recorded. The test provides an assessment of the extrinsic clotting pathway, i.e. factors I (fibrinogen), II (prothrombin), V, VII and X. Common causes of a prolonged PT are listed in Table 16.2.

To facilitate the comparison of results between laboratories, PT results are often converted into an 'International Normalised Ratio' result (INR). The higher the result, the longer it takes for blood to clot.

ACTIVATED PARTIAL THROMBOPLASTIN TIME (APTT)

Different chemicals are added to a blood sample, and the time taken to clot is recorded. This test provides an assessment of the intrinsic clotting pathway, i.e. all clotting factors except factor VII. Table 16.3 lists causes of a prolonged APTT.

A common source of confusion occurs when blood is sampled from a central line that has been 'locked' with heparin. In such situations, it is necessary to withdraw and discard a sample before collecting blood for

Test	Abbreviation
Prothrombin time	PT
Activated partial thromboplastin time	APTT
Fibrinogen	–

Table 16.1   *The component parts of a coagulation screen*

Cause	Notes
Deficiency of relevant clotting factor	–
Drugs	For example, warfarin
Liver failure	An excellent test in acute liver failure as clotting factors have a short half life
Vitamin K deficiency	–
Disseminated intravascular coagulation	This in itself has a variety of causes

Table 16.2   *Causes of a prolonged prothrombin time*

Cause	Notes
Deficiency of relevant clotting factor	For example, haemophilia A (factor VIII deficiency)
Drugs	For example, heparin
Vitamin K deficiency	–
Disseminated intravascular coagulation	This in itself has a variety of causes.

Table 16.3   *Causes of a prolonged activated partial thromboplastin time*

analysis. If this is not done, heparin-contaminated blood will be sampled, and a falsely elevated APTT will be reported.

FIBRINOGEN

Fibrinogen is the precursor for fibrin, a key component of blood clots. In the disorder with most extreme clotting (disseminated intravascular coagulation, DIC), very low levels of fibrinogen are expected.

Deep venous thrombosis
Pulmonary embolism
Recent surgery or trauma
Pregnancy
Inflammatory process
Cancer

Table 16.4   *Common causes of a raised D-dimer*

D-DIMER

When the body makes a clot, the fibrinolytic system begins to dissolve it. So-called 'fibrinogen degradation products' can be measured, D-dimer being the most common. D-dimer is most commonly tested when a venous thrombo-embolic event (e.g., deep venous thrombosis or pulmonary embolism) is suspected. Whilst the D-dimer has a high negative predictive value (i.e. a clot is unlikely if D-dimer is low), its positive predictive value is less impressive (i.e. a positive result does not guarantee that a clinically significant clot is present). Causes of a raised D-dimer are shown in Table 16.4.

OTHER TESTS

Thrombin time (TT)

Thrombin is added to a blood sample, and the time taken to clot is recorded. A prolonged TT is found in patients with fibrinogen disorders and in those receiving heparin.

Coagulation correction tests

If a patient's PT, APTT or TT is prolonged, but normalises when 'healthy' plasma is added to the sample, the implication is that the patient's plasma is lacking in one or more clotting factors. If this process makes no difference to the clotting, the sample may contain an abnormal inhibitor of coagulation.

Clotting factor tests

It is possible to measure the concentration of individual clotting factors to identify deficiencies.

103

Platelet count and platelet function testing

Platelets play a key role in blood clotting. The platelet count is provided as part of the full blood picture. Platelet function testing can be undertaken in some circumstances.

CHAPTER 17

Blood grouping

When it comes to blood grouping and transfusion, very little interpretation is required by the test requestor, as clear reports are produced that can simply be read off. Haemovigilance procedures are well established to reduce the chance of a patient receiving a transfusion of a blood product meant for someone else. It is imperative that proper procedures are followed when requesting a blood group test. In particular, blood bottles must not be labelled in advance of taking the sample for fear of sample mix-up. A basic description of blood groups is provided here to assist you in interpreting these reports.

There are several hundred blood groups in existence, but the most important group to understand is the 'ABO' system. Imagine that circulating red blood cells have 'labels' on their surfaces. People with blood group A have the 'A' label, those with blood group B have 'B' labels. AB patients have both 'A' and 'B', and those with group O blood have no such labels. Next, you should understand that patients have circulating antibodies to labels that they do not normally possess. If they receive a blood transfusion containing cells with these labels on their surfaces, these antibodies will attack the 'foreign' blood and a transfusion reaction will occur. This is summarised in Fig. 17.1.

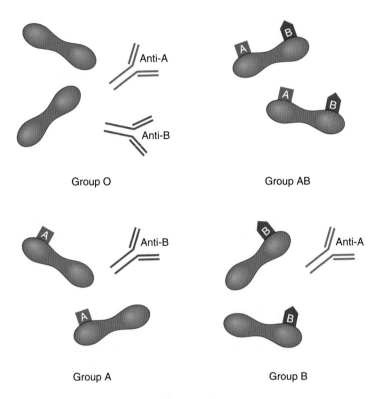

Group O

Group AB

Group A

Group B

Fig. 17.1 *A simple representation of the ABO blood grouping system*

Case studies and self-assessment questions

CHAPTER 1

Case study

A 50-year-old woman, who has no significant medical history, pays privately for a series of 'health screening tests'. As part of this, she undergoes several blood tests and is found to have a very slightly raised amylase level. Concerned that there might be something wrong with her pancreas, she then chooses to undergo a computed tomography scan of her abdomen. This scan reveals a normal pancreas but shows a nodule on the left adrenal gland. She is informed that she has a mass on one of the adrenal glands and is referred to an endocrinologist for an opinion. In the meantime, she conducts research about adrenal tumours and convinces herself that she has cancer. After a very anxious wait, she undergoes a series of specialised blood tests and urine collections. Finally, she is informed that no abnormalities have been identified, and it is likely that the nodule on the adrenal gland is an incidental finding and nothing to be concerned about.

This case illustrates how finding an abnormal test result can result in a series of investigations which can be very costly and generate considerable anxiety. Always request tests that are clinically justifiable and be careful about putting undue emphasis on a result which is unexpected or just outside the reference range.

Self-assessment 1

A hospital chest pain clinic has a point-of-care device installed for the analysis of troponin (a marker of heart damage). Which of the following is an advantage of using this technology over sending a sample to the hospital laboratory for analysis?
a) Faster speed of analysis
b) Less training required
c) More robust analysis
d) Reduction in test cost

Self-assessment 2

Which of the following laboratory techniques is most used in the analysis of a blood sample for the presence of ethylene glycol (antifreeze)?
a) Chromatography
b) Electrophoresis
c) Mass spectrometry
d) Potentiometry

Self-assessment 3

A laboratory scientist is concerned that a particular test result is falsely low because of the 'high-dose hook' effect. What might the scientist do to a sample to detect this problem?
a) Centrifuge the sample at high speed
b) Dilute the sample
c) Evaporate water from the sample to make it more concentrated
d) Refrigerate the sample overnight and analyse the next day

Self-assessment 4

Which of the following laboratory techniques is most used for the measurement of the sodium concentration in a urine sample?
a) Microscopy
b) Osmometry
c) Potentiometry
d) Spectrophotometry

CHAPTER 2

Case study

A young woman is brought to the emergency department after a seizure. She is unresponsive, and limited details are available. Needle track marks are noted on her arms, so it is suspected that she is an intravenous drug user. Venepuncture is extremely difficult, but after several attempts, a small sample of blood is obtained. Point-of-care testing reveals hyperkalaemia, with a potassium level of 6.7 mmol/L. No electrocardiogram changes of hyperkalaemia are noted, but the team treat her elevated potassium with calcium gluconate, insulin, and dextrose. Shortly afterwards, a central line is inserted, and a venous blood sample is sent to the laboratory for electrolyte analysis. The result shows mild hypokalaemia with a level of 3.3 mmol/L. The initial sample was haemolysed, and the potassium result of 6.7 mmol/L was erroneous. Because the point-of-care analyser does not check for haemolysis, this was not appreciated, and the patient was treated unnecessarily.

Self-assessment 1

Which of the following blood sample types does not contain clotting factors?
a) Capillary blood
b) Plasma
c) Serum
d) Whole venous blood

Self-assessment 2

A patient in a vascular surgery ward is noted to have a significant drop in their blood creatinine concentration following a procedure. Their kidney function was normal beforehand. Which procedure is likely to have been carried out?
a) Abdominal aortic aneurysm repair
b) Amputation of lower limb
c) Femoral-popliteal arterial bypass
d) Varicose vein stripping

Self-assessment 3

After a difficult venepuncture, many of the biochemical tests requested for a patient are not reportable due to the degree of haemolysis in the sample. Which of the following tests is particularly affected by haemolysis?
a) Albumin
b) Alkaline phosphatase
c) Creatinine
d) Potassium

Self-assessment 4

An unexpectedly high lithium result is returned for a patient who is taking a very low dose of lithium for bipolar disorder. Inappropriate use of a tube of which cap colour might account for this finding?
a) Gold
b) Green
c) Grey
d) Purple

CHAPTER 3

Case study

A patient recovering from elective hip surgery is found to have new, significant hyponatraemia 3 days postoperatively. The ward doctor examines the patient and finds them to be euvolaemic. She orders a range of investigations which are returned as follows:

Test	Patient result	Reference range
Sodium	122 mmol/L	136-145 mmol/L
Potassium	5.1 mmol/L	3.5-5.3 mmol/L
Chloride	92 mmol/L	95-108 mmol/L
CO_2	24 mmol/L	22-29 mmol/L
Urea	7.7 mmol/L	2.5-7.8 mmol/L
Creatinine	82 µmol/L	45-84 µmol/L
Estimated glomerular filtration rate (eGFR)	>60 mL/min/1.73 m²	>60 mL/min/1.73 m²
Serum osmolality	258 mosmol/kg	275-295 mosmol/kg
Urinary sodium	64 mmol/L	No reference range
Urinary osmolality	621 mosmol/kg	No reference range

Since the serum osmolality is low, the hyponatraemia is genuine; this is not pseudohyponatraemia. The urinary sodium result was greater than 30 mmol/L, making dehydration unlikely, and is in keeping with the clinical impression of volume status. The urine is much more concentrated than the serum. This may be caused by drugs, renal failure, hypothyroidism, hypoadrenalism, or syndrome of inappropriate antidiuretic hormone secretion (SIADH).

The patient begins to complain of a headache and nausea. The doctor is concerned that these symptoms are because the patient is developing cerebral oedema. A bolus of hypertonic saline is administered. A repeat sample 30 minutes after administration reveals that the serum sodium has risen to 126 mmol/L, and the patient's symptoms resolve quickly. The cause turned out to be SIADH, most likely related to postoperative pain.

Self-assessment 1

A patient's results reveal the following: sodium 155 mmol/L, potassium 3.8 mmol/L, chloride 102 mmol/L, total carbon dioxide 24 mmol/L, urea

12.2 mmol/L, creatinine 240 μmol/L, and glucose 5.4 mmol/L. What is the calculated osmolality?
a) 274.6 mmol/L
b) 335.2 mmol/L
c) 352.8 mmol/L
d) 542.4 mmol/L

Self-assessment 2

A patient with congestive cardiac failure is on long-term treatment with bisoprolol, ramipril, furosemide, and spironolactone. They develop acute kidney injury after a severe episode of gastroenteritis. Which of the following electrolyte abnormalities is most likely in this scenario?
a) Hyperkalaemia
b) Hypernatraemia
c) Hypokalaemia
d) Hyponatraemia

Self-assessment 3

An inpatient in a psychiatric unit has their urea and electrolyte profile checked and is found to be hyponatraemic. Serum osmolality is low. A urine sample is sent for analysis and is found to have an osmolality of 89 mosmol/kg. The patient is found to be clinically euvolaemic. What is the most likely cause of the hyponatraemia?
a) Hypoadrenalism
b) Liver failure
c) Primary polydipsia
d) SIADH

Self-assessment 4

A patient in the emergency department is found to have hyperkalaemia when blood is analysed using a point-of-care device. A fresh blood sample is sent to the laboratory, and the potassium result comes back normal. What is the most likely explanation for this discrepancy in results?
a) Acute kidney injury
b) Familial hyperkalaemic periodic paralysis
c) Haemolysis of the point-of-care sample
d) Incorrect calibration of the point-of-care analyser

CHAPTER 4
Case study

A 65-year-old man presents with generalised lethargy. A bone profile is organised as part of a battery of tests and reveals the following:

Test	Patient result	Reference range
Calcium	3.74 mmol/L	2.20-2.60 mmol/L
Phosphate	1.32 mmol/L	0.80-1.50 mmol/L
Alkaline phosphatase (ALP)	578 U/L	30-130 U/L
Albumin	39 g/L	35-50 g/L
Adjusted calcium	3.80 mmol/L	2.20-2.60 mmol/L

The parathyroid hormone concentration is below the threshold for detection. Renal function and thyroid function are normal, and the vitamin D concentration is in the 'sufficient' range. An isotope bone scan is performed and shows appearances in keeping with widespread bony metastases. A prostatic specific antigen (PSA) test supports the diagnosis of advanced prostate cancer. He is referred to a urologist for a prostate biopsy before being referred for chemotherapy.

Self-assessment 1

A middle-aged woman who is known to abuse alcohol presents after a fall. She is found to have severe hypomagnesaemia. Which of the following electrolyte disturbances is likely to be associated with this?
a) Hyperkalaemia
b) Hypocalcaemia
c) Hyperphosphataemia
d) Hyponatraemia

Self-assessment 2

A patient complains of muscle cramps and undergoes a bone profile. Calcium is 1.86 mmol/L and albumin 25 g/L. What is the adjusted calcium?
a) 1.46 mmol/L
b) 1.56 mmol/L
c) 2.16 mmol/L
d) 2.26 mmol/L

Self-assessment 3

A 72-year-old man complains of marked deep-seated bony pain in the upper left arm and mid right thigh. Blood tests reveal:

Test	Patient result	Reference range
Calcium	2.42 mmol/L	2.20-2.60 mmol/L
Phosphate	0.91 mmol/L	0.80-1.50 mmol/L
ALP	391 U/L	30-130 U/L
Albumin	41 g/L	35-50 g/L
Adjusted calcium	2.50 mmol/L	2.20-2.60 mmol/L

What is the likely cause of the pain?
a) Osteomalacia
b) Paget's disease of bone
c) Primary hyperparathyroidism
d) Psychosomatic

Self-assessment 4

A woman with a history of breast cancer is found to have mild hypercalcaemia. A parathyroid hormone level is checked as part of preliminary investigations.

Test	Patient result	Reference range
Parathyroid hormone	61 pg/mL	15-65 pg/mL

What is the most likely explanation for the hypercalcaemia?
a) Bony metastases
b) Hyperthyroidism
c) Primary hyperparathyroidism
d) Tuberculosis

CHAPTER 5

Case study

A 56-year-old man is found to have abnormal liver enzymes. He denies drinking alcohol, has no risk factors for viral hepatitis, and has not been taking prescribed or other drugs. An ultrasound scan of his liver is performed, but no abnormalities are seen. His general practitioner (GP) sends a full panel of screening tests. His iron profile reveals a grossly elevated ferritin and a transferrin saturation of 59%. Genetic testing reveals that he is homozygous for the C282Y mutation on the *HFE* gene, in keeping with hereditary haemochromatosis. He undergoes regular venesection, and his liver tests return to normal after several months.

Self-assessment 1

A man is recovering in hospital following a crush injury to his leg. He has myoglobinuria and acute kidney injury. The attending team check liver enzymes and are concerned to find that the aspartate aminotransferase (AST) concentration is moderately raised. What is the likely explanation?

a) Cholestasis
b) Hepatitis
c) Macro-AST
d) Rhabdomyolysis

Self-assessment 2

A 40-year-old woman is admitted with jaundice. Tests reveal the following:

Test	Patient result	Reference range
Bilirubin	112 µmol/L	<21 µmol/L
ALT	621 U/L	<33 U/L
ALP	154 U/L	30-130 U/L
AST	567 U/L	<32 U/L
GGT	163 U/L	6-42 U/L
Albumin	41 g/L	35-50 g/L

What is the most likely cause of the jaundice?
a) Gallstones
b) Haemolysis
c) Paracetamol toxicity
d) Viral hepatitis

Self-assessment 3

A 62-year-old man is referred to a medical clinic for investigation of abnormal liver tests. He has no medical history of note, takes no medication, and claims to not drink alcohol. Immunoglobulins are checked as part of his investigations and reveal the following:

Test	Patient result	Reference range
IgG	7.9 g/L	6.0-16.0 g/L
IgA	6.2 g/L	0.8-4.0 g/L
IgM	0.8 g/L	0.5-2.0 g/L

What is the most likely cause of his problems?
a) Alcohol
b) Coeliac disease
c) Autoimmune hepatitis
d) Primary biliary cirrhosis

Self-assessment 4

A 25-year-old woman has blood checked as part of an insurance medical. Liver testing reveals the following:

Test	Patient result	Reference range
Bilirubin	48 μmol/L	<21 μmol/L
ALT	31 U/L	<33 U/L
ALP	52 U/L	30-130 U/L
AST	14 U/L	<32 U/L
GGT	35 U/L	6-42 U/L
Albumin	43 g/L	35-50 g/L

Which test would be helpful in providing an explanation for the abnormality seen?
a) α-1 antitrypsin
b) Caeruloplasmin
c) Reticulocyte count
d) Transferrin saturation

CHAPTER 6

Case study

A 62-year-old woman with moderately severe chronic obstructive pulmonary disease is reviewed at the respiratory clinic. She is reasonably well controlled. An arterial blood gas analysis reveals the following:

115

Test	Patient result	Reference range
pH	7.41	7.35-7.45
P_aO_2	9.2 kPa	11.0-14.0 kPa
P_aCO_2	6.5 kPa	4.5-6.0 kPa
Bicarbonate	41 mmol/L	22-26 mmol/L

Two weeks later, she is admitted to hospital with an infective exacerbation. She is acutely breathless and has been coughing up green sputum. Blood gas testing now reveals the following:

Test	Patient result	Reference range
pH	7.28	7.35-7.45
P_aO_2	8.8 kPa	11.0-14.0 kPa
P_aCO_2	7.1 kPa	4.5-6.0 kPa
Bicarbonate	42 mmol/L	22-26 mmol/L

Despite good care, her condition deteriorates, and she becomes drowsy. Another blood gas sample is obtained:

Test	Patient result	Reference range
pH	7.21	7.35-7.45
P_aO_2	9.1 kPa	11.0-14.0 kPa
P_aCO_2	8.5 kPa	4.5-6.0 kPa
Bicarbonate	40 mmol/L	22-26 mmol/L

She is commenced on non-invasive ventilation and responds well. After 4 hours, her blood gas results are as follows:

Test	Patient result	Reference range
pH	7.35	7.35-7.45
P_aO_2	9.2 kPa	11.0-14.0 kPa
P_aCO_2	6.8 kPa	4.5-6.0 kPa
Bicarbonate	41 mmol/L	22-26 mmol/L

Self-assessment 1

A woman who appears to be in her 30s is brought to the resuscitation room by ambulance having been found collapsed in the street. They are not on supplemental oxygen. Arterial blood gas analysis reveals the following:

Test	Patient result	Reference range
pH	6.97	7.35-7.45
P_aO_2	12.2 kPa	11.0-14.0 kPa
P_aCO_2	2.8 kPa	4.5-6.0 kPa
Bicarbonate	4 mmol/L	22-26 mmol/L
Sodium	142 mmol/L	136-145 mmol/L
Potassium	5.9 mmol/L	3.5-5.3 mmol/L
Chloride	95 mmol/L	95-108 mmol/L
CO_2	5 mmol/L	22-29 mmol/L
Urea	8.9 mmol/L	2.5-7.8 mmol/L
Creatinine	130 µmol/L	45-84 µmol/L
eGFR	49 mL/min/1.73 m²	>60 mL/min/1.73 m²

What is the most likely explanation for her presentation?
a) Acute renal failure
b) Diabetic ketoacidosis
c) Paracetamol poisoning
d) Renal tubular acidosis

Self-assessment 2

A 58-year-old man with motor neurone disease becomes increasingly unwell. They are not on supplemental oxygen. Arterial blood gas analysis reveals the following:

Test	Patient result	Reference range
pH	7.15	7.35-7.45
P_aO_2	7.8 kPa	11.0-14.0 kPa
P_aCO_2	9.7 kPa	4.5-6.0 kPa
Bicarbonate	35 mmol/L	22-26 mmol/L

Which is the correct description of the acid-base disturbance?
a) Metabolic acidosis
b) Metabolic alkalosis
c) Respiratory acidosis
d) Respiratory alkalosis

Self-assessment 3

A patient recovering from surgery is noted to have a low total CO_2 result on routine testing and has an arterial blood gas sample taken to further investigate. They are not on supplemental oxygen. The results are as follows:

Test	Patient result	Reference range
pH	7.29	7.35-7.45
P_aO_2	13.2 kPa	11.0-14.0 kPa
P_aCO_2	3.9 kPa	4.5-6.0 kPa
Bicarbonate	15 mmol/L	22-26 mmol/L
Sodium	137 mmol/L	136-145 mmol/L
Potassium	3.9 mmol/L	3.5-5.3 mmol/L
Chloride	110 mmol/L	95-108 mmol/L
CO_2	15 mmol/L	22-29 mmol/L
Urea	2.6 mmol/L	2.5-7.8 mmol/L
Creatinine	52 µmol/L	45-84 µmol/L
eGFR	>60 mL/min/1.73 m^2	>60 mL/min/1.73 m^2

What is the most likely cause of the acid-base disturbance?
a) High output stoma
b) Lactic acidosis
c) Starvation ketoacidosis
d) Type 4 renal tubular acidosis

Self-assessment 4

A patient complains of shortness of breath and the following arterial blood gas results are returned. They are not on supplemental oxygen.

Test	Patient result	Reference range
pH	7.50	7.35-7.45
P_aO_2	13.5 kPa	11.0-14.0 kPa
P_aCO_2	1.9 kPa	4.5-6.0 kPa
Bicarbonate	25 mmol/L	22-26 mmol/L

Which is the most likely explanation for these results?
a) Exacerbation of chronic obstructive pulmonary disease
b) Hyperammonaemia
c) Primary hyperventilation
d) Vomiting

CHAPTER 7

Case study

A 51-year-old man undergoes investigations for generalised lethargy. An electrolyte profile shows mild hyponatraemia and hyperkalaemia, so he undergoes adrenal testing. The 9 am cortisol level is low, and an urgent Short Synacthen test is arranged. The results are as follows:

Time	Cortisol (nmol/L)	Reference range (nmol/L)
0	42	166 – 507
30 mins	72	>420

The Synacthen test confirms hypoadrenalism. The adrenocorticotropic hormone level is inappropriately low, so secondary hypoadrenalism is deemed likely. A further panel of tests revealed a slightly low thyroxine level with normal thyroid-stimulating hormone (TSH; secondary hypothyroidism); low testosterone, luteinising hormone (LH), and follicle-stimulating hormone (FSH; secondary hypogonadism); and low IGF-1 (due to growth hormone deficiency). Prolactin is raised. Brain imaging confirms the presence of a pituitary tumour. Appropriate hormone replacement is arranged, and he is referred for pituitary surgery.

Self-assessment 1

A 42-year-old man presents with erectile dysfunction. As part of his workup, his GP requests a male sex hormone profile. Results from a 9 am blood draw are as follows, and similar results are obtained when the tests are repeated:

	Patient result	Reference range
Testosterone	3.1 nmol/L	8.6-29.0 nmol/L
FSH	39.1 IU/L	1.5 – 12.4 IU/L
LH	25.2 IU/L	1.7-8.6 IU/L

Which of the following is a likely cause for this presentation?
a) Autoimmune hypophysitis
b) Depression
c) Pituitary tumour
d) Previous mumps infection

Self-assessment 2

A patient with newly diagnosed atrial fibrillation has her thyroid function checked. Free thyroxine is grossly elevated and TSH is suppressed. Which

test result is most strongly associated with an underlying diagnosis of Graves' disease?
a) Anti-thyroglobulin antibody
b) Anti-thyroid peroxidase antibody
c) Elevated erythrocyte sedimentation rate
d) TSH receptor antibody

Self-assessment 3

Which of the following factors would not be expected to yield a spuriously high blood cortisol level?
a) Alcohol ingestion
b) Exercise
c) Long-term prednisolone treatment
d) Psychological stress

Self-assessment 4

A young woman with severe hypertension is investigated to identify an underlying cause and is eventually diagnosed with primary hyperaldosteronism. What clue to this diagnosis is often present?
a) Hyperprolactinaemia
b) Hypokalaemia
c) Hyponatraemia
d) Renal impairment

CHAPTER 8

Case study

A 68-year-old woman is found to have osteoporosis after sustaining a fragility fracture of her hip. Bone densitometry reveals markedly discrepant readings in the areas examined, so she is referred for further assessment. A skeletal survey shows multiple lytic lesions throughout the skeleton. Serum protein electrophoresis reveals a large IgG-κ paraprotein band and an excess of κ free light chains is confirmed on measurement of free light chains. A working diagnosis of multiple myeloma is made, and she is referred to a haematologist for treatment. Further testing reveals several complications of myeloma: calcium is high, she is anaemic, and has renal impairment.

Self-assessment 1

A woman is referred to a rheumatology clinic with suspected systemic sclerosis. Which autoantibody should be checked?
a) Anti-Jo-1
b) Anti-parietal cell
c) Anti-scleroderma-70
d) Cytoplasmic-anti-neutrophil cytoplasmic

Self-assessment 2

An 85-year-old man undergoes a panel of investigations when he is found to be anaemic. Selected results are shown below.

Sodium	141 mmol/L	136-145 mmol/L
Potassium	3.9 mmol/L	3.5-5.3 mmol/L
Chloride	100 mmol/L	95-108 mmol/L
CO_2	25 mmol/L	22-29 mmol/L
Urea	6.8 mmol/L	2.5-7.8 mmol/L
Creatinine	51 µmol/L	45-84 µmol/L
eGFR	>60 mL/min/1.73 m^2	>60 mL/min/1.73 m^2
Bilirubin	15 µmol/L	<21 µmol/L
ALT	31 U/L	<33 U/L
ALP	118 U/L	30-130 U/L
AST	30 U/L	<32 U/L
GGT	38 U/L	6-42 U/L
Albumin	35 g/L	35-50 g/L
Total protein	105 g/L	60-80 g/L

Which investigation should be requested next?
a) Anti-tissue transglutaminase antibody
b) Vitamin B_{12} and folate
c) Iron profile
d) Serum protein electrophoresis

Self-assessment 3

A specialist osteoporosis physician monitors procollagen 1 amino-terminal extension peptide (P1NP) in a patient at high risk of fracture. Baseline and on-treatment levels are 87 and 28 ng/mL, respectively. Which of the following are in keeping with this trend?
a) Anabolic treatment effect
b) Anti-resorptive treatment effect

c) Impaired renal function
d) Recent fracture

Self-assessment 4

An 18-year-old man is admitted with rhabdomyolysis after attempting a half marathon with no training. Which of the following features should prompt consideration of an underlying metabolic disorder?
a) A previous similar episode
b) Creatine kinase >10× the upper limit of normal
c) No similar episodes in family members
d) Persistent rise of creatine kinase beyond 5 days

CHAPTER 9

Case study

A 65-year-old man attends his GP complaining of excessive thirst and passing more urine than normal. A non-fasting point-of-care glucose recording is 10.5 mmol/L, and an oral glucose tolerance test is requested for the next morning. This reveals a fasting glucose of 7.5 mmol/L and a 2-hour post-test glucose of 15.2 mmol/L, so a diagnosis of diabetes mellitus is made. HbA1c is 76 mmol/mol. He opts to try to improve his diet, lose weight, and exercise more. After 3 months, HbA1c has improved to 68 mmol/mol. His GP then commences metformin; after a further 3 months, HbA1c is down to 55 mmol/L and his symptoms are much improved.

Self-assessment 1

A middle-aged woman undergoes an oral glucose tolerance test. Results are as follows:

	Time 0	Time 2 hours
Glucose	5.8 mmol/L	8.1 mmol/L

What is the correct characterisation of glycaemic status?
a) Diabetes mellitus
b) Impaired fasting glucose
c) Impaired glucose tolerance
d) Normal

Self-assessment 2

An infant is found to be hypoglycaemic, and a panel of investigations are ordered. Which disorder should be considered after consideration of the following results?

	Time 0
Glucose	1.8 mmol/L
3-Hydroxybutyrate	<0.03 mmol/L

a) Galactosaemia
b) Hypoadrenalism
c) Medium-chain acyl CoA dehydrogenase deficiency
d) Phenylketonuria

Self-assessment 3

A 52-year-old man is admitted for investigations into recurrent hypo-glycaemia. The following results are obtained during a hypoglycaemic episode 18 hours into a fast:

Glucose	2.5 mmol/L	Random, 4.0-8.0 mmol/L
Insulin	39 mU/L	Fasting, 2.6-24.9 mU/L
C-peptide	6.8 µg/L	1.1-4.4 µg/L

What is the most likely diagnosis?
a) Exogenous insulin administration
b) Hypoadrenalism
c) Insulinoma
d) Liver failure

Self-assessment 4

A patient with sickle-cell anaemia is diagnosed with type 2 diabetes. Which of the following tests should be used for monitoring long-term control?
a) Fructosamine
b) Glucose
c) HbA1c
d) Insulin

CHAPTER 10
Case study

A 28-year-old man is worried about his health after his older brother suffered a myocardial infarction at age 35 years. On further enquiry, his doctor discovers that his mother developed angina in her late 40s and went on to have coronary artery bypass grafting performed. His maternal aunt died from a myocardial infarction in her 50s. On examination, the doctor finds thickened Achilles tendons in keeping with tendon xanthomata, and a lipid profile is obtained. This shows the following:

Cholesterol	9.7 mmol/L	<5 mmol/L
Triglyceride	1.20 mmol/L	<1.7 mmol/L
High-density lipoprotein (HDL)	1.2 mmol/L	>1 mmol/L
Low-density lipoprotein (LDL)	7.8 mmol/L	<3 mmol/L
Chol/HDL Ratio	8.1	-
Non-HDL-cholesterol	8.5 mmol/L	- mmol/L

Genetic testing reveals that he is heterozygous for a common mutation in the gene encoding the LDL receptor, so a diagnosis of heterozygous familial hypercholesterolaemia is made. He is offered lifestyle advice and lipid-lowering therapy, and 1 year later his LDL is down to 2.5 mmol/L. Cascade screening is arranged so that the wider family can be tested for the condition.

Self-assessment 1

Which of the following lipid parameters conveys a favourable cardiovascular risk when present in relatively high amounts?
a) Apolipoprotein A-1
b) Lipoprotein (a)
c) LDL cholesterol
d) Non-HDL cholesterol

Self-assessment 2

Which of the following lipid parameters forms part of the QRISK3 cardiovascular risk tool?
a) Apolipoprotein B
b) Cholesterol:HDL cholesterol ratio
c) LDL cholesterol
d) Non-HDL cholesterol

Self-assessment 3

Patients with which of the following lipid disorders would be expected to have a creamy layer floating on plasma when their blood sample is refrigerated overnight?
a) Dysbetalipoproteinaemia
b) Familial chylomicronaemia syndrome
c) Familial hypercholesterolaemia
d) Polygenic hypercholesterolaemia

Self-assessment 4

Which of the following conditions would not be expected to cause a rise in cardiac troponin?
a) Aortic dissection
b) Myocardial infarction
c) Pulmonary embolism
d) Stable angina

CHAPTER 11

Case study

An 82-year-old man is diagnosed with localised prostate cancer and is treated with androgen deprivation therapy. His PSA is 20.2 ng/mL at the time of diagnosis, but after 6 months falls to 0.5 ng/mL. He is followed by an oncologist at regular intervals for three years and his PSA is consistently less than 1 ng/mL. He then has an admission to hospital with severe community-acquired pneumonia and is admitted to the intensive care unit for supportive care. He is discharged after 4 weeks in hospital and is reviewed by his oncologist shortly after. The PSA on this occasion is raised at 7.6 ng/mL and it is supposed that this might have been related to the insertion of a urinary catheter when he was unwell. However, a further PSA check after 4 weeks shows a rising level at 10.2 ng/mL; further detailed imaging of the prostate is arranged and additional treatment is offered.

Self-assessment 1

A patient is concerned about getting their PSA tested. Which of the factors below would not be expected to raise PSA?
a) Digital rectal examination
b) Family history of prostate cancer
c) Prostate cancer
d) Vigorous exercise

Self-assessment 2

A 40-year-old woman is found to have a slightly high cancer antigen (CA)-125 level. There is no sign of ovarian cancer on imaging. Which of the following is not a recognised cause for this result?
a) Endometriosis
b) Irritable bowel syndrome
c) Pelvic inflammatory disease
d) Pregnancy

Self-assessment 3

What of the following is a vital characteristic of a tumour marker?
a) High positive predictive value
b) High sensitivity
c) Long half-life
d) Low specificity

Self-assessment 4

A patient with alcoholic cirrhosis is regularly screened for hepatocellular carcinoma. Which tumour marker will be requested for this purpose?
a) α-Foetoprotein
b) 5-Hydroxyindoleacetic acid
c) Chromogranin-A
d) CA-15-3

CHAPTER 12

Case study

A man in his 50s undergoes complex small bowel surgery after a flare of Crohn's disease. His body mass index is low, and his nutritional state is poor. His team wish to commence parenteral nutrition to aid his recovery but are very concerned about him developing re-feeding syndrome. Measures of potassium, magnesium, calcium, and phosphate are found to be normal prior to the commencement of feeding, which is started at a very slow rate. Twenty-four hours later, the phosphate and magnesium levels are found to fall. Intravenous replacement of both phosphate and magnesium is provided, and the rate of feeding slowed further. After a further 48 hours of slow feeding and electrolyte replacement, blood levels of these substances normalise. The patient has ongoing bowel complications, and parenteral nutrition is continued for several weeks. The team arrange a full nutritional screen during this timeframe so that deficiencies can be corrected.

Self-assessment 1

A 21-year-old woman is found to be anaemic. Which of the following features would suggest iron deficiency as a possible cause?
a) High ferritin
b) High lactate dehydrogenase level
c) High mean cell volume
d) High total iron binding capacity

Self-assessment 2

A middle-aged woman is found to have slightly abnormal enzymes. Her doctor sends off a large panel of liver investigations and is concerned about Wilson's disease when a slightly high blood copper level is detected. Which of the following can cause a high copper level?
a) Copper intra-uterine device
b) Oral contraceptive pill
c) Working as a jeweller
d) Zinc supplementation

Self-assessment 3

A patient with vague neurological symptoms is found to have a borderline-low vitamin B_{12} level. Which of the following test results would be supportive of true B_{12} deficiency as a cause of the symptoms?
a) High holotranscobalamin
b) High methylmalonic acid
c) Low folate
d) Low total homocysteine

Self-assessment 4

A 72-year-old man with multiple medical problems is found to have a very low blood magnesium concentration. Which of the following drugs is most likely to be responsible?
a) Aspirin
b) Carbamazepine
c) Lansoprazole
d) Spironolactone

CHAPTER 13
Case study

An elderly man is brought to the emergency department in a state of collapse. His Glasgow Coma Scale score is 8/15 but he is haemodynamically stable. Initial blood test results are shown below:

Test	Patient result	Reference range
pH	7.04	7.35-7.45
P_aO_2	13.1 kPa	11.0-14.0 kPa
P_aCO_2	1.8 kPa	4.5-6.0 kPa
Bicarbonate	6 mmol/L	22-26 mmol/L
Lactate (point-of-care)	2.1 mmol/L	0.5-2.2 mmol/L

Test	Patient result	Reference range
Sodium	140 mmol/L	136-145 mmol/L
Potassium	5.6 mmol/L	3.5-5.3 mmol/L
Chloride	101 mmol/L	95-108 mmol/L
CO_2	7 mmol/L	22-29 mmol/L
Urea	25.3 mmol/L	2.5-7.8 mmol/L
Creatinine	657 µmol/L	45-84 µmol/L
eGFR	7 mL/min/1.73 m^2	>60 mL/min/1.73 m^2
Glucose	4.1 mmol/L	Random, 4.0-8.0 mmol/L
Serum osmolality	357 mosmol/kg	275-295 mosmol/kg
Lactate (Laboratory)	8.2 mmol/L	0.5-2.2 mmol/L

His attending team note the profound metabolic acidosis and work out the anion gap to be raised at 32 mmol/L. The discrepancy between the point-of-care and laboratory lactate results are also noted (lactate gap). The estimated osmolality is 320.6 mosmol/kg, which is significantly lower than that measured in the lab – this is a significant osmolar gap. The on-call biochemist undertakes analysis for toxic alcohols, and the presence of significant quantities of ethylene glycol is confirmed. Treatment with fomepizole (an antidote) and haemodialysis are commenced in the intensive care department.

Self-assessment 1

Which of the following antimicrobial drugs routinely require therapeutic drug monitoring to guide dosing?
a) Amoxicillin
b) Ciprofloxacin
c) Metronidazole
d) Vancomycin

Self-assessment 2

A patient is being treated for paracetamol poisoning. At presentation, 5 hours post-ingestion, the paracetamol level was well above the treatment line. The team repeat the paracetamol level after a further 5 hours and it is now below the treatment line. Which is the most appropriate action?
a) Continue treatment
b) Measure coagulation before deciding on continuing treatment
c) Measure liver enzymes before deciding on continuing treatment
d) Stop treatment

Self-assessment 3

Which of the following acid-base disturbances is most in keeping with mild salicylate toxicity?

Test	Reference range
pH	7.35-7.45
P_aCO_2	4.5-6.0 kPa
Bicarbonate	22-26 mmol/L

a) pH 7.48, P_aCO_2 3.4 kPa, Bicarbonate 25 mmol/L
b) pH 7.27, P_aCO_2 8.8 kPa, Bicarbonate 35 mmol/L
c) pH 6.19, P_aCO_2 1.5 kPa, Bicarbonate 8 mmol/L
d) pH 7.50, P_aCO_2 5.8 kPa, Bicarbonate 42 mmol/L

Self-assessment 4

Which of the following factors is a predictor of poor outcome in patients with digoxin toxicity?
a) Hypercalcaemia
b) Hyperkalaemia
c) Hypomagnesaemia
d) Hyponatraemia

129

CHAPTER 14

Case study

An obese woman who has struggled to lose weight for many years travels abroad to have bariatric surgery performed. She has surgical complications post-surgery, and a further operation is performed. All is initially well following her return home, but she is subsequently admitted to hospital three times with episodes of confusion and lethargy. On the most recent of these, an arterial blood gas analysis is performed and reveals the following:

Test	Patient result	Reference range
pH	7.27	7.35-7.45
P_aO_2	12.1 kPa	11.0-14.0 kPa
P_aCO_2	3.2 kPa	4.5-6.0 kPa
Bicarbonate	13 mmol/L	22-26 mmol/L
Lactate	1.9 mmol/L	0.5-2.2 mmol/L

The anion gap is raised, but renal function and ketones are normal. Specialised testing confirms a significant concentration of D-lactic acid and a diagnosis of D-lactic acidosis secondary to altered bowel anatomy is made.

Self-assessment 1

A 35-year-old woman has a history of recurrent episodes of severe hyperammonaemia. Her twin brother died in infancy, but no satisfactory cause of death was provided at the time. What is the likely explanation for the elevated ammonia?

a) Citrullinaemia
b) Liver failure
c) Ornithine transcarbamylase deficiency
d) Propionic acidaemia

Self-assessment 2

A patient has been admitted several times in the last few years with acute abdominal pain but, despite extensive investigations, no cause for her presentations has been found. On her latest admission, a junior doctor decides to test urinary porpholinogen, and the level is found to be markedly raised. What is the likely diagnosis?

a) Acute intermittent porphyria
b) Hereditary coprophorphyria

c) Porphyria cutanea tarda
d) Variegate porphyria

CHAPTER 15

Case study

An elderly woman complains of severe headache and scalp tenderness on the right side of her head. Her GP is concerned about the possibility of temporal arteritis and requests an urgent test of erythrocyte sedimentation rate (ESR). The result is very high at 105 mm/h. The patient is treated with high-dose steroids, and her symptoms settle over the course of a few days. A re-check of ESR 2 weeks later shows that it has fallen to 45 mm/h, and it is 21 mm/h after another 4 weeks. The steroid dose is gradually tapered over the course of several months, but 3 months later the woman phones to say that she is feeling unwell, and a similar headache has returned. ESR is found to be 88 mm/h, so the doctor advises that the steroid dose is immediately increased again.

Self-assessment 1

A patient with anaemia is found to have a deficiency of iron, folate, and vitamin B_{12}. Which red cell index might give a clue to the multifactorial nature of the anaemia?
a) Haematocrit
b) Mean cell haemoglobin
c) Red blood cell count
d) Red cell distribution width

Self-assessment 2

A 20-year-old woman from Libya is diagnosed with iron-deficiency anaemia. Three months after commencing iron supplements, she is found to have the following results:

	Pre-iron	Post-iron	
Hb	68 g/L	74 g/L	115-165 g/L
Mean cell volume	62 fL	64 fL	76-100 fL

What test would be most useful next?
a) Haemoglobin electrophoresis
b) Holotranscobalamin

131

c) Red cell folate
d) Soluble transferrin receptors

Self-assessment 3

A man who works in a glass foundry is found to have lead toxicity. Which of the following blood film abnormalities is characteristic?
a) Anisocytosis
b) Basophilic stippling
c) Pappenheimer bodies
d) Target cells

Self-assessment 4

An elderly man with severe chronic obstructive pulmonary disease is found to have an elevated haematocrit. What is the most likely explanation?
a) Chronic hypercarbia
b) Deficiency in vitamin B_{12}
c) Elevated erythropoietin
d) Polycythaemia rubra vera

CHAPTER 16

Case study

A 32-year-old woman who is 30 weeks pregnant is involved in a car collision and sustains blunt trauma to her abdomen. By the time of arrival in the local hospital, she is experiencing abdominal pain and vaginal bleeding. A diagnosis of placental abruption is made. Her clinical condition deteriorates during transfer to an obstetric centre. An urgent coagulation screen check is made upon arrival in that centre and shows the following:

Prothrombin time	29.2 s	10-13 s
Activated partial thromboplastin time	61.9 s	24-38 s
Fibrinogen	0.4 g/L	2-5 g/L

A diagnosis of disseminated intravascular coagulation is made, and she receives urgent blood product support pending obstetric surgery.

Self-assessment 1

Which of the following tests provides the most rapidly changing indicator of synthetic liver function in a patient with acute liver failure?
a) Activated partial thromboplastin time
b) Fibrinogen
c) Prothrombin time
d) Thrombin time

Self-assessment 2

Two very different coagulation profile results are returned on a patient in the intensive care unit. The samples are timed 5 minutes apart, but the results are very different. A repeat profile is arranged. Which of the following is not a valid explanation for the difference in results obtained?
a) One same tube underfilled
b) One sample contaminated with heparin in central line
c) One tube is from another patient and has been mislabelled
d) The patient takes warfarin, and the international normalised ratio has been erratic

CHAPTER 17

Self-assessment 1

A military field hospital is dealing with large numbers of trauma victims, and a shortage of blood products soon arises. Persons with which blood group are considered to be 'universal donors'?
a) A Rhesus positive
b) AB Rhesus negative
c) B Rhesus positive
d) O Rhesus negative

Self-assessment: answers

CHAPTER 1

Self-assessment 1: a) Faster speed of analysis
Self-assessment 2: a) Chromatography
Self-assessment 3: b) Dilute the sample
Self-assessment 4: c) Potentiometry

CHAPTER 2

Self-assessment 1: c) Serum
Self-assessment 2: b) Amputation of lower limb
Self-assessment 3: d) Potassium
Self-assessment 4: b) Green

CHAPTER 3

Self-assessment 1: b) 335.2 mmol/L
Self-assessment 2: a) Hyperkalaemia
Self-assessment 3: c) Primary polydipsia
Self-assessment 4: c) Haemolysis of the point-of-care sample

CHAPTER 4

Self-assessment 1: b) Hypocalcaemia
Self-assessment 2: d) 2.16 mmol/L
Self-assessment 3: b) Paget's disease of bone
Self-assessment 4: c) Primary hyperparathyroidism

CHAPTER 5

Self-assessment 1: d) Rhabdomyolysis
Self-assessment 2: d) Viral hepatitis
Self-assessment 3: a) Alcohol
Self-assessment 4: c) Reticulocyte count

CHAPTER 6

Self-assessment 1: b) Diabetic ketoacidosis
Self-assessment 2: c) Respiratory acidosis
Self-assessment 3: a) High-output stoma
Self-assessment 4: c) Primary hyperventilation

CHAPTER 7

Self-assessment 1: d) Previous mumps infection
Self-assessment 2: d) TSH receptor antibody
Self-assessment 3: c) Long-term prednisolone treatment
Self-assessment 4: b) Hypokalaemia

CHAPTER 8

Self-assessment 1: c) Anti-scleroderma-70
Self-assessment 2: d) Serum protein electrophoresis
Self-assessment 3: b) Anti-resorptive treatment effect
Self-assessment 4: a) A previous similar episode

CHAPTER 9

Self-assessment 1: c) Impaired glucose tolerance
Self-assessment 2: c) Medium-chain acyl CoA dehydrogenase deficiency
Self-assessment 3: c) Insulinoma
Self-assessment 4: a) Fructosamine

CHAPTER 10

Self-assessment 1: a) Apolipoprotein A-1
Self-assessment 2: b) Cholesterol:HDL cholesterol ratio
Self-assessment 3: b) Familial chylomicronaemia syndrome
Self-assessment 4: d) Stable angina

CHAPTER 11

Self-assessment 1: b) Family history of prostate cancer
Self-assessment 2: b) Irritable bowel syndrome
Self-assessment 3: b) High sensitivity
Self-assessment 4: a) α-Foetoprotein

CHAPTER 12

Self-assessment 1: d) High total iron binding capacity
Self-assessment 2: b) Oral contraceptive pill
Self-assessment 3: b) High methylmalonic acid
Self-assessment 4: c) Lansoprazole

CHAPTER 13

Self-assessment 1: d) Vancomycin
Self-assessment 2: a) Continue treatment
Self-assessment 3: a) pH 7.48, P_aCO_2 3.4 kPa, Bicarbonate 25 mmol/L
Self-assessment 4: b) Hyperkalaemia

CHAPTER 14

Self-assessment 1: c) Ornithine transcarbamylase deficiency
Self-assessment 2: a) Acute intermittent porphyria

CHAPTER 15

Self-assessment 1: d) Red cell distribution width
Self-assessment 2: a) Haemoglobin electrophoresis
Self-assessment 3: b) Basophilic stippling
Self-assessment 4: c) Elevated erythropoietin

CHAPTER 16

Self-assessment 1: c) Prothrombin time
Self-assessment 2: d) The patient takes warfarin, and the international normalised ratio has been erratic

CHAPTER 17

Self-assessment 1: d) O Rhesus negative

Index

Page numbers followed by '*f*' indicate figures and '*t*' indicate tables.